NEW ASPECTS OF VENTRICULAR ASSIST DEVICES

Edited by **Guillermo Reyes**

New Aspects of Ventricular Assist Devices
Edited by Guillermo Reyes

Published by InTech

Janeza Trdine 9, 51000 Rijeka, Croatia

Publishing Process Manager Iva Lipovic

Technical Editor Teodora Smiljanic

Cover Designer InTech Design Team

Additional hard copies can be obtained from orders@intechopen.com

New Aspects of Ventricular Assist Devices, Edited by Guillermo Reyes
p. cm.
ISBN 978-953-307-676-8

Meet the editor

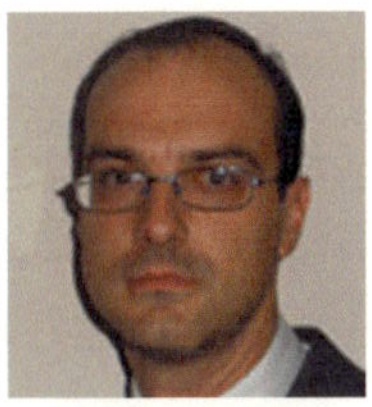

Dr. Reyes, MD, PhD is currently working as a cardiac surgeon in La Princesa Hospital in Madrid, Spain, which he joined in 2005 and become chief resident. He completed medical school training in Lyon, France and visited several centres in United States of America to complete his formation. He obtained his PhD degree in 2005 with a thesis concerning the use of the radial artery in CABG surgery. He has one Master in Statistics and one Master in Administration and Direction of Health Systems. He has published many articles in different journals, including studies regarding the use of VADs and is a member of the reviewer committee of several journals. He has been the Principal Investigator of many clinical trials and the first surgeon combining TMR therapy with stem cells injection in Europe. He has also been training cardiac surgeons from other institutions in Spain and internationally on this advanced revascularization therapy. He is specialized in doing cardiac surgery without the use of blood products, being a national reference for the management of patients requiring bloodless surgery.

Contents

Preface

Ventricular assist devices are the future, but also the present. They are meant not only to increase the survival of patients, but also to improve their quality of life. The technology that involves these devices improves every year. It is essential not only to choose the right patient for a VAD implantation, but also to know when is the right time to do it.

It is very important to be updated about the advances in VAD technology, the physiopathology of the assisted heart and the outcomes of patients who receive this therapy. Now VADs are available for short, intermediate and long term support. This means that a wide spectrum of patients may benefit from this therapy. The associated complications following the use of VAD will be reduced with the use of more modern devices, a better understanding of the physiopathology of the assisted heart and a better patient selection.

Numerous international authors have participated in the creation of this book. We have compiled their experience and their concern about ventricle assist device therapy. In order to organize the book content two sections have been created. First part will focus on aspects concerning how the heart will behave when a VAD is implanted and some new aspects regarding VAD technology. Secondly, clinical outcomes and others aspects of patients are updated and commented in different ways.

I would like to thank especially the authors of this book. They have shared their experience, knowledge and time with all of us. To care for patients and spread our knowledge may be sometimes the first step to achieve our goal.

Dr. Guillermo Reyes
Department of Cardiovascular Surgery
La Princesa University Hospital, Madrid
Spain

Part 1

Physiopathology of Ventricular Assist Devices

1

Importance of Arterial Conduit Function Assessment in Chronic Congestive Heart Failure: Predictors of True Circulatory Decompensation for Optimal Timing of Mechanical Circulatory Support

Henryk Siniawski and Roland Hetzer
Department of Cardiothoracic and Vascular Surgery,
Deutsches Herzzentrum Berlin,
Germany

1. Introduction

Circulatory failure with no reaction to medical treatment requires urgent mechanical circulatory support to save the patient's life and to open up the way for broader medical options. When ventricular assist devices (VAD) must be urgently implanted in patients suffering not only from hemodynamic shock but from the disastrous consequences of prolonged hypoperfusinon of vital organs, they are associated with high mortality. Good early and late outcome can be anticipated by the principle "good patient, good outcome." In this sense a "good patient" for assist device implantation is one in whom the surgical procedure is undertaken in optimal time and not after the "zone of death" is reached, when the patient is suffering from multiorgan failure. Unfortunately optimal means of prognostic assessment of patients suffering from chronic circulatory failure are lacking. The available clinical guidelines are rather opened as a "road map" for the treatment until the treatment response is blunted and it is necessary to turn to the next step on this road.

From our viewpoint it is necessary to distinguish between diagnostic means of helping to assess or even predict the transition from chronic compensated to acutely decompensated heart failure and the assessment of various factors as predictors of mortality. In other words acute precipitants such as rising left ventricular filling pressure, pulmonary rales etc. and physical signs[1] of congestive heart failure or even precipitants reflecting the conversion from a chronic compensated to a decompensated pathophysiological state do not necessarily help to set the indication for assist device implantation. These established factors today still lack reliability. The decompensation which "suddenly appears easy to treat" indicates that even acute worsening of chronic heart failure can be managed successfully by medical means. The important issue is to predict the risk of "true decompensation" (decompensation resistant to conventional treatment). The assessment of such factors is very valuable for estimating the optimal time-point for the implantation of mechanical circulatory support. Finding the optimal time also means that univentricular (usually left ventricular) support may be sufficient. In such cases the outcome is better than with extracorporeal support of both ventricles.

The goal of assessment of the "circulatory reserve" of the individual patient suffering from chronic circulatory failure is important; however the issue is very complicated. Until now such "factors" are unknown. More studies are needed to put together all known factors and, on the basis of statistical analysis, to extract "significant predictors influencing mortality." There are several problems that should be taken into account here.

Recent studies have suggested a multifactorial model containing many risk factors with statistical definition of their importance. The multifactorial risk model makes sense when the risk factors are correctly identified; otherwise, imprecise and misleading information can cloud the issue. The concept of setting a model with statistically prepared multirisk factors [2] as a "check list" is difficult to accept practically in clinical settings. Even separating the risks into precisely identified groups or goals (precipitating and predisposing) does not help clinicians to identify the best form of preventive intervention.

By critical examination of such a multifactorial model at least the following conclusions have to be drawn: The systolic function of the left ventricle is no longer of value in predicting survival of the patients when profound systolic dysfunction has occurred[3,4]. The dynamic development of congestive heart failure (<12 month period)[5] is an important factor; however in the less malignant course the number of episodes of decompensation is truly important. Laboratory tests (sodium[6], BNP[7], noradrenalin level[8]) can help to identify individual patients possibly characterized by low reserve compensation mechanisms. The function of the right heart chamber and pulmonary pressure are factors that predict mortality, but their practical value - their value for the prediction of the life expectancy - is limited[9,10]. Continuous ambulatory monitoring on the basis of telemetric data transmitted by miniaturized technology[11] of the right-sided pressures[12] (for example the value of pulmonary pressure at time of closure of the pulmonary valve corresponds to the left filling pressure) can be used to detect the transition to decompensation and are therefore valuable in predicting risk (SENSE-HF trial,[13] CLEPSYDRA[14]). Continuous telemetric hemodynamic monitoring does not assess the circulatory reserves directly but rather informs the clinician that the physiological balance of the hemodynamics inside the circulation as a whole system has broken down. New criteria that could precisely predict the clinical state of the patients are badly needed to make the surgical decision for optimal timing of mechanical support in chronically ill patients.

To understand the subject it is necessary to review the changing viewpoints on congestive heart failure. Congestive heart failure means chronic "circulatory failure" or "heart failure," caused, for example, by end-stage dilated cardiomyopathy.

1.1 Historical resumé

The quality of the arterial pulse was first described as early as the sixteenth century by the Polish physician Josephus Struthius in his work *Sphygmicae artis* (published in Basel in 1555). His knowledge of the pulse is still utilized today (e.g. the distinction between pulsus altus, parvus, rarus, celler and durus) and is used not only to diagnose a heart pathology such as mitral stenosis or aortic incompetence but also for heart failure staging. Traditional understanding of systolic heart failure was based on invasive investigation performed on the basis of animal studies performed in 1879 in Berlin,[15] and diastolic function assessment was undertaken at the beginning of the last century.[16] Heart function was regarded as of central importance on the way to understanding the pathology of circulation since the beginning of the era of modern medicine but the importance of the "circulation" was also pointed out. The state of "heart failure" was described in Latin as "stadio circulatoria suffitientiae relativae" or "circulatioria in stadio insuffitiantiae," corresponding to the English expression, "congestive heart failure." Traditionally the meaning of "congestion" was reserved exclusively for the venous vascular bed. Nevertheless, in addition to myocardial failure, circulatory congestion was taken to be an important part of the phenomenon called "heart failure." The role of the "peripheral" circulation was seemingly forgotten.

Nowadays the vascular resistance, as the representation of the circulation and especially of conduit physiology, appears rather more as a hemodynamic result of the heart function and the arterial system response. It is usually defined as the force of opposition known as "resistance" but not as an active and important functional unit that cooperates actively with the heart. However, the researchers and physicians dealing with mechanical circulatory support are recognizing the problem of circulatory failure but rather only semantically, writing of "mechanical circulatory support in heart failure." Unfortunately this recognition is usually limited to expression and does not incorporate evidence-based medical factors of the importance of the circulation.

1.2 Changing concept of the failing heart

Reduction of left atrial loading conditions (preload) significantly alters the diastolic transmitral pressure relation and thus profoundly affects the Doppler flow velocity profile.[17] On the other hand the afterload also influences heart function. It is important to know how afterload affects preload in order to define the function of the extracardiac circulatory system. A.C. Guyton stated in 1955: "When a change occurs in the hemodynamics of the circulation system one cannot predict what will happen to the cardiac output unless to take in consideration both the effect of this change on the ability of the heart to pump blood and also on the tendency for blood to return to the heart from the blood vessels"[18].

This research produced a "volume pressure curve" of the systemic arterial and venous compartment which documents the interplay between venous pressure and volume in arterial and venous segments in dependence on stimulation or inhibition[19]. On the other hand the venous return influences the atrial pressure and consequently cardiac output (Guyton diagrams)[20], not to forget that venous return is regulated by the arterial system.

Briefly, the pumping ability of the heart depends mostly on the venous return if the diseased heart is in stable condition after a destructive process has been healed. It should be stated that not the worsening of the failing myocardiac function but rather circulatory dysfunction during the chronic phase is the cause of worsening of the circulation as a whole.

The monitoring of the arterial and venous compartment can help to define the hemodynamic condition and find predictors of the final event of decompensation.

The arterial part of the circulation (arterial conduit) is easy to access and, being situated between the venous compartment and heart function, not only has the passive function of conduction of the blood but is an active part of the circulation.

In normal human beings the heart can mobilize reserves so that the cardiac output can rise five times, for example from 6 l/min to 30 l/min in athletes. The severely diseased heart is hardly able to raise cardiac output by more than 10%. The arterial tree can change the distribution of perfusion, depending on the acute need, to supply the more important organs and let other organs "hibernate." The physiological process known as "preconditioning" is responsible for the smoothly functioning economy of the body with a constant lack of oxygen. The circulation, and especially the arterial compartment, demonstrates abnormal vascular response to volume unloading when the heart is failing.[21] This implies that the arterial conduit is responsible for decompensation and is the key to stabilizing the circulation and to describing diagnostically its function and dysfunction. Virtually speaking there is the level of arterial conduit dysfunction beyond which compensation is not possible; below these levels "true" decompensation is only a matter of time. This concept of congestive heart failure is the clue to understanding the transition from the compensated to the decompensated state in patients suffering from heart failure.

1.3 Arterial conduit function

The left ventricle mechanically loads the systemic circulation in a pulsated manner. In abnormal LV function the circulation is supplied under special conditions determined by the autonomic properties of the vascular bed.

The influence of the arterial system on the heart as a pump in congestive heart failure is seldom presented in the literature; it is more often studied as its own unit of interest that responds to different deconditioning mechanisms.[22,23,24] Although the importance of pulse and blood pressure is always studied in hypertensive patients, the relation between the effect of the left chamber work, defined as stroke, and the arterial tree has not been adequately recognized. This may be the essential key to heart failure pathophysiology.

There are several methods of defining the active operation of the arterial conduit (large and small resistance arteries) interacting directly with the heart ejection. One of the simplest and most commonly applied to determine the stage of cooperation between the heart and the arterial system is invasive or non-invasive measurement of pressure in one of the branches of the arterial system. The pressure measured is the main criterion for diagnosis of acute heart failure (vasoactive shock). In recent years the importance of systolic pressure as a predictor of mortality in patients with acute and chronic[25] forms of heart failure has been recalled. Low pressure in patients suffering from chronic forms of heart failure is recognized as a positive prognostic factor of mortality. However, the explanation of this phenomenon is based rather on a monotheory that failure of the heart (low cardiac output) may play a first role[26] (partial truth), but not that dysfunction of the arterial conduit - as an interactive organ - may also be involved in the state of "circulatory failure." Nevertheless there exists agreement that the result of interaction of the heart and arterial conduit - blood pressure - is an important prognostic factor for assessing the risk of mortality in acute and chronic forms of "heart failure."

Additional information on the circulatory state may be based on investigation of the relationship between cardiac output and blood pressure by a formula called the "cardiac power"[27] or "circulatory power" during peak exercise in stable patients.[28] The pumping power of the heart is determined as the product of cardiac output (simultaneously measured) and mean arterial pressure.

A study of patients suffering from acute forms of heart failure, especially those with ejection fraction of below 40%, has documented that systolic blood pressure was linearly and inversely associated with mortality.[27]

1.3.1 Windkessel model

Any part of the cardiovascular system, when it is compliant, possesses a volume reserve according to needs. The arterial windkessel model is based on a "system of tubes" as a representation of the arterial tree and allows analysis of the resistance and compliance of the arterial conduit.

1.3.2 Pressure-flow analyses in the time domain

Accurate non-invasively measured central arterial pressure and flow in large arteries available for investigation (e.g. the carotid artery) can be used for pressure-flow analysis. Using computational equipment to analyze both signals (pressure and flow) gives unique possibilities to assess interaction of the diseased heart and the arterial conduit. One method based on this principle is wave intensity (WI) measurement.

2. Wave intensity

The concept of wave intensity is based on simultaneous computerized analysis of the blood ejected into the arterial conduit, which causes the phenomenon of interaction of flow (the velocity of the stroke volume) with the flow mechanics inside the studied vessel and the interaction of pressure and compliance of the vessel. The simultaneous study of flow and pressure interaction enables WI assessment.

To understanding the whole concept it is necessary to review shortly the basic physiology of heart ejection as a function of the whole circulation. The early phase of ejection is characterized by a positive pressure gradient in the left ventricular outflow tract (LVOT) and a rise in both pressure and flow in the ascending aorta. After this phase the pressure still rises but the flow falls. During approximately the last third of ejection there is a negative pressure gradient in the LVOT and ejection persists, while flow and pressure fall until the aortic valve closes. Ejection occurs because the momentum of the blood shifts the last part of the stroke against higher pressure above the aortic valve.

It has to be remembered that the pressure difference between the LVOT and ascending aorta is negative late in systole (during 2nd wave building). The ejection of blood into the aorta during this time results from the momentum of the ejected blood.[29] This phase is characterized by gentle relaxation of the myocardium[30] - leading to a smooth return of the muscle function from contraction to relaxation. The effect of this cooperation "gently" stops the back blood flow (before aortic valve closure) and again it should be stated that the relation of flow and pressure is directly related to the blood momentum but also to the diastolic quality of the heart muscle, which defines diastolic function of the heart before aortic valve closure (traditionally taken as the event signalling the relaxation period).

Invasive wave intensity (WI) index is well described by Parker et al.[31] and is primarily calculated from invasive parameters as the product of the derivatives of the simultaneously measured pressure and velocity inside the artery:

$$WI = (dP/dt) \bullet (dV/dt)$$

where P= pressure and V= flow.

The non-invasive simultaneous analysis of pressure change and flow signals sampled during short constant intervals (5 ms) can be used for real-time non-invasive WI (NWI) analysis.

The waveform of carotid wall displacement (dU) closely corresponds to pressure change (dP) in a carotid artery measured invasively with high correlation quotient (goodness of fit $r^2=0.97$) and can be substituted for the invasively recorded pressure waveform.[32] This study by Sugawara et al. has opened up the way to the assessment of NWI, because high fidelity pressure and flow signals are easily obtainable by ultrasonic investigation. Non-invasive wave intensity (NWI) is defined on the basis of echocardiography[33] (ALOKA Ultrasonic System, Japan). The formula for NWI is as follows:

$$NWI = (dU/dt) \bullet (dV\ Doppler/dt)$$

where dU = difference in displacement of carotid artery and V = flow velocity measured by Doppler.

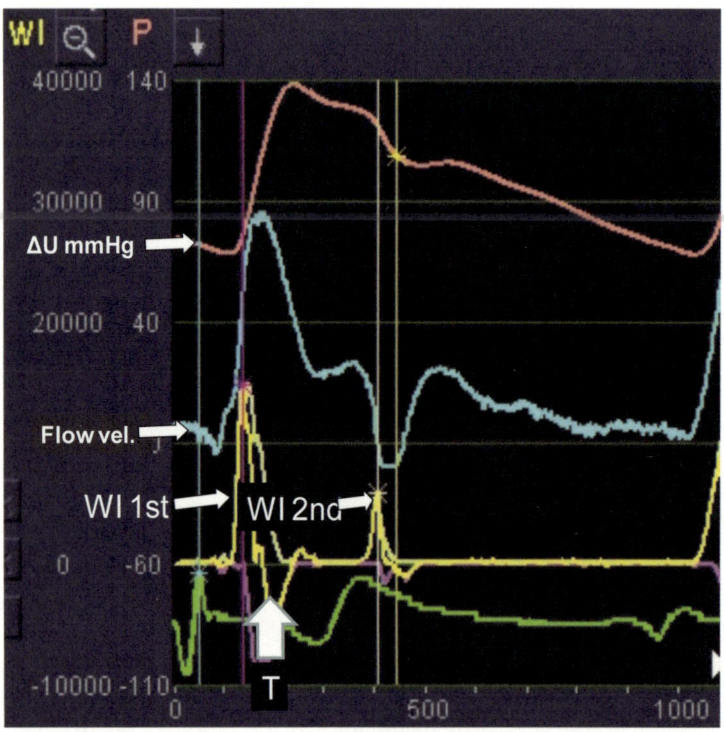

Fig. 1. The noninvasive WI index assessed in a normal subject. The yellow curve of WI consists of two peaks (1st and 2nd). The 1st peak is the "compression wave" and the 2nd peak the "expansion" wave. The pressure (red curve) is marked "ΔU mmHg" and flow waveform (green curve) "flow vel.". The wave T is marked by a white arrow

The NWI index materializes as the curve consisting of two mathematically defined peaks (1st and 2nd). The 1st peak is the "compression wave" and is mathematically positive as a product of two positive values of first derivatives of pressure and flow waveform as demonstrated mathematically (Fig. 1). The compression wave of the 1st peak of WI describes the state of myocardial contractility of the LV in relation to the afterload. At the end of isovolumic contraction (which is the beginning of the 1st peak) the LV pressure becomes equal to aortic diastolic pressure which indicates that the LV begins to challenge the afterload force.[34] The height of the peak is directly related to LV contractility and to stroke volume at a given afterload. This parameter reflects very tiny differences in ejection dynamics and stroke volume (at given/constant afterload) and can be used as a marker of circulatory reserves but also as a versatile marker in many clinical situations. The 2nd peak is created during the negative pressure gradient in the LVOT and is influenced by the momentum of the blood ejected into the aorta. The value of momentum of blood ejection in the last phase of ejection is connected to relaxation of the LV. Simplifying the physiological dispute, this means that during ejection the blood is stopped by the gentle slowing of the LV ejection during the last part of ejection (when the pressure in the LV chamber is lower than in the aorta), which reflects the idea of relaxation of the LV myocardium, as was experimentally documented by Solomon.[35] This explains why the 2nd peak is related to the relaxation of the myocardium which begins before aortic valve closure.

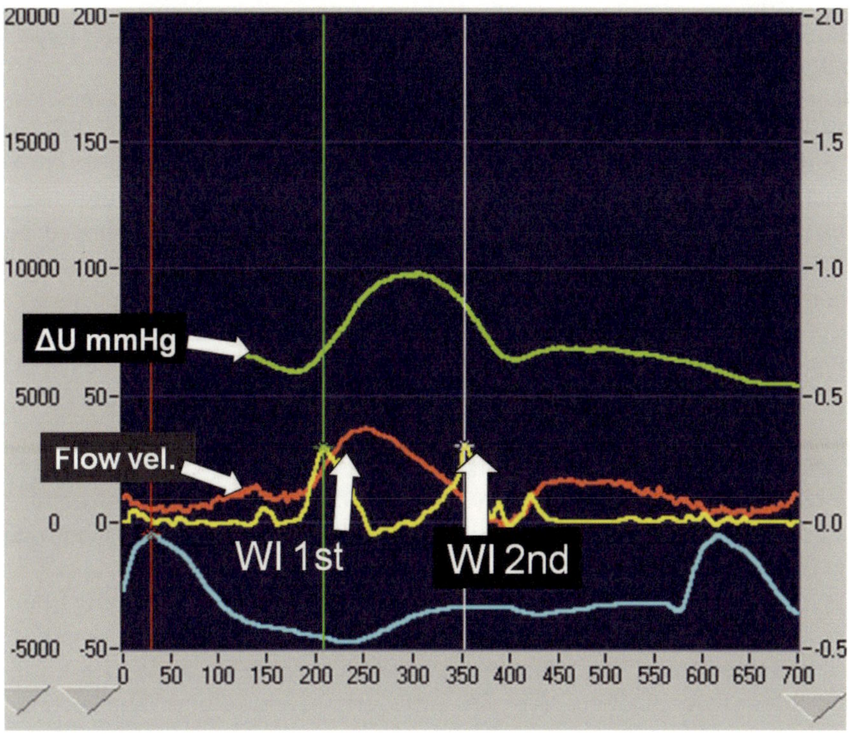

Fig. 2. The noninvasive WI (yellow curve) from a patient suffering from end-stage dilated cardiomyopathy during "true decompensation". Note that the green curve represents pressure and the red curve represents flow

Returning to the second phase of ejection, it is necessary to describe the negative part of WI appearing as the continuation of the 1st peak and named negative T wave (Fig. 1). The T wave is formed by the negative product of pressure and flow (dU / dt) • (dV / dt) where pressure is still rising and flow is diminishing (mixed mathematical factors reflected as negative product).

During WI investigation several parameters are obtainable: negative area T, arterial stiffness as beta value (β), diameter of the artery studied, minimal and maximal flow in the artery

and dynamic changes in real time of several other parameters. The T wave was not found to have prognostic importance in our studies.
The 2nd peak of WI ("expansion wave") is calculated in the same way as the 1st peak, which means that it is the result of algebraically calculated pressure and flow inside the vessel after ejection. While both curves (pressure and flow) in this phase are negative, algebraically their derivates produce a positive 2nd peak of WI. In general this peak defines diastolic function of the heart (active relaxation of the myocardium in systole) and the diastolic function of the conduit (elastic properties, filling of the conduit, which is similar to LV filling). The 2nd peak is usually smaller than the 1st but in pulsus alternans or in a situation of passively overfilled arterial conduit (with any kind of rotary pump support) it can be higher than the 1st peak if the heart possesses native ejection.

2.1 Human studies

2.1.1 Influence of alternant beat (reduced contractility) on wave intensity (type A pathology of myocardial failure)

The pathophysiology of pulsus alternans is diverse and there are several theories that are used to explain this phenomenon. Although description of all these theories is not necessary for this purpose, it is important to note that the majority of considerations are based on myocardial, electrical and hemodynamic functional components. The myocardial theory is based on the alteration of diastolic prosperities of myocytes of the diseased heart[36,37], whereas the electrical alternans theory[38] is based on the primary alteration of electrical stimulation, secondarily influencing myocardial reaction. The hemodynamic theory explains "weak beats" on the basis of worse filling of the chamber (loading conditions) and alteration of the Frank-Starling curve. Independently of different theories that could explain the pathology of pulsus alternans the one beat is strong ("normal" for studied individual) and the second is weak. In other words the stroke volume is alternately normal and smaller, causing normal pulse quality, and the second beat is weak and recognizable on the blood pressure curve or by studying the pulse in any other way. It is well documented that pressure in late diastole rises more slowly in the weak beat, which has to interpreted by an alteration in diastolic compliance[39].
Figures 3 A and B demonstrate WI applied in an ambulatory patient suffering from DCM at the stage of NYHA III and having pulsus alternans (3B). WI peaks from "strong" (3A) and "weak" (3B) beats identify the hemodynamics of the composite of the heart and arterial conduit in this individual. The 1st (Fig. 3A, white arrow) and second WI peak (Fig. 3A, red arrow of the "strong beat" are typical findings in heart failure patients. The 1st WI peak is small but the 2nd peak is relatively higher than in normal individuals and is responsible for the quotient of relation of the 1st to the 2nd peak being 2:1 (1st 3441 to 2nd 1834 mmHg*s^3), whereas in normal persons it is usually 6:1.
The second beat is "weak" and is produced by suboptimal stroke volume (Fig. 3B) influencing the pulse curve peak (P) which is smaller and rises more slowly. The simultaneously recorded flow (F) curve also rises more slowly, so that the 1st peak of WI as a product of the derivatives of pressure/flow (dU/ dt) • (dV / dt) is reduced to 50% of the previous strong beat. The 2nd peak is preserved and both peaks are at the level of 1800 mmHg*s^3. The high 2nd peak of WI is exemplified by a negative and sharp fall in the product of the derivatives pressure and flow recorded simultaneously. An explanation of the reduction of the 1st and preservation of the 2nd

peak of WI helps us to understand the importance of WI as a tool defining hydraulic cooperation of the arterial conduit and the heart. The lower and less "dynamic" the early ejection phase, the lower the 1st peak for given compliance of the conduit is. The 2nd peak of WI illustrates and defines the level of the conduit filling (see next subsection), the value of ejected blood momentum during the 3rd phase of ejection, and compliance of the chamber at the end of systole before aortic valve closure. This 2nd peak is inversely related to diastolic compliance of the LV and inversely related to the state of filling of the conduit (see below).

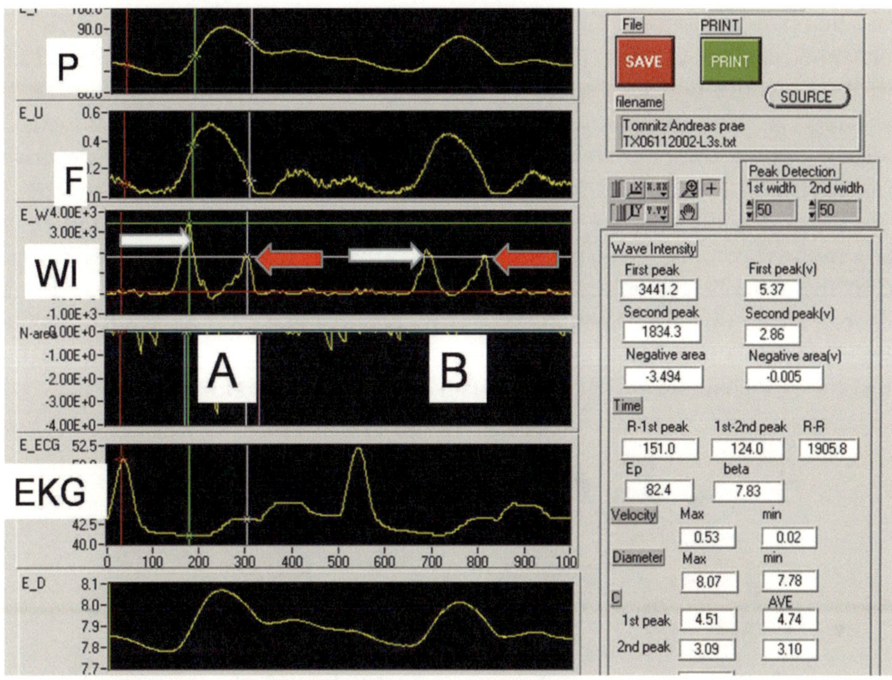

Fig. 3. Noninvasive WI in a patient suffering from end-stage dilative cardiomyopathy who has pulsus alternans. A: strong beat; B: weak beat. P= pressure curve. F= flow curve. White arrow 1st and red arrow 2nd peak of WI. EKG= electrocardiogram

2.1.2 Mixed pathology of arterial volume overloading and systolic heart dysfunction influences wave intensity (type B pathology)

The clinical picture of congestive heart failure when arterial congestion is present can be illustrated by the case of a patient who suffered from acute myocardial infarction complicated by cardiogenic shock 7 days after successful revascularization during Impella mechanical circulatory support (Fig. 4A). This is a schematic representation of arterial filling during Impella support with flow of 3.5 l/min and native stroke volume of the heart of only 20 ml. Because the LV chamber is partially unloaded (filling pressure only 7 mmHg) the stroke volume is low and reaches only the level of 20 ml. The 1st peak is low (approx. 5500 mmHg*s^3) and produced by slowly rising pressure and simultaneous slowly rising flow curve during the first phase of systole (Fig. 5A). The 2nd peak is high (approx. 8800 mmHg*s^3) and produced by sharply falling pressure and flow (even below the zero line) during the last phase of systole. The diameter of the artery was significantly larger than during reduced Impella flow (6.93±1.39 vs. 6.45±1.97 mm respectively, $p = 0.003$). Reduced systolic function of the diseased heart and unloading defined by the Starling principle reflect type 1 pathology ("weak" beat of pulsus alternans) and is responsible for low 1st peak. The 2nd peak of WI is not proportionally higher, reflecting severe diastolic dysfunction and arterial overloading. During the procedure of weaning from Impella there are important alterations in the loading conditions of the heart and arterial conduit (Fig. 4B). In this stage, when the pump did not significantly fill the arterial conduit (0.2 l/min) the patient was treated with high doses of epinephrine and the heart was driven by adequate filling for this state of disease (PCP 18 mmHg), producing stroke volume of 40 ml.

The value and relations of peaks during spontaneous heart function (with maximal Impella support the heart did not possess sufficient filling to eject) is presented in Fig. 5B. The 1st peak was high (approx. 21,000 mmHg*s^3.) after medical support and the second was higher than normal (approx. 3800 mmHg*s^3). High 2nd peak can be explained by high negative flow in the conduit and a rapid fall in the pressure curve before aortic valve closure. These phenomena are mainly due to rapid vanishing of the value of momentum of blood, reflecting reduced compliance of the heart muscle after infarction. The 2nd peak is inversely related to the diastolic compliance of the LV (and all parameters influencing myocardial compliance). Again this experimental study demonstrates that 1st peak is related to systolic function of the heart in relation to arterial conduit function. The 2nd peak defines diastolic function of the LV chamber and the filling state of the arterial conduit.

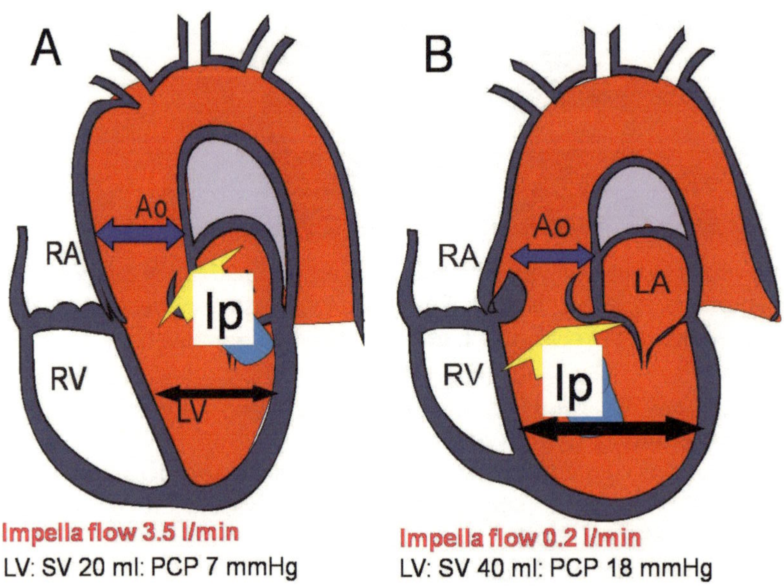

Fig. 4. Schematic drawing of the heart chambers and aorta (Ao) during different stages of seventh day Impella support in a patient following successful surgical revascularization, suffering from heart infarction complicated by cardiogenic shock. A: Impella (Ip) low 3.5 l/min (stage A); B: Impella flow (Ip) 0.2 l/min (stage B). Blue arrows indicate aortic dimension (Ao) dependent on Impella support. Black arrows indicate LV dimension dependent on Impella support. LA = left atrium, RA = right atrium, RV = right ventricle, SV = stroke volume, PCP = pulmonary capillary pressure

Physiological cooperation between the chambers and the arterial conduit means that under a given filling pressure of both sides adequate systolic performance is maintained in changing circumstances (resistance, preload, afterload) which can be monitored noninvasively by WI. One can hypothesize that these two types of pathology (A, primary myocardial dysfunction and B, myocardial dysfunction and volume shift into the arterial conduit, responsible for congestion) are probably the icons of the daily clinical situations in patients suffering from end-stage congestive heart failure.

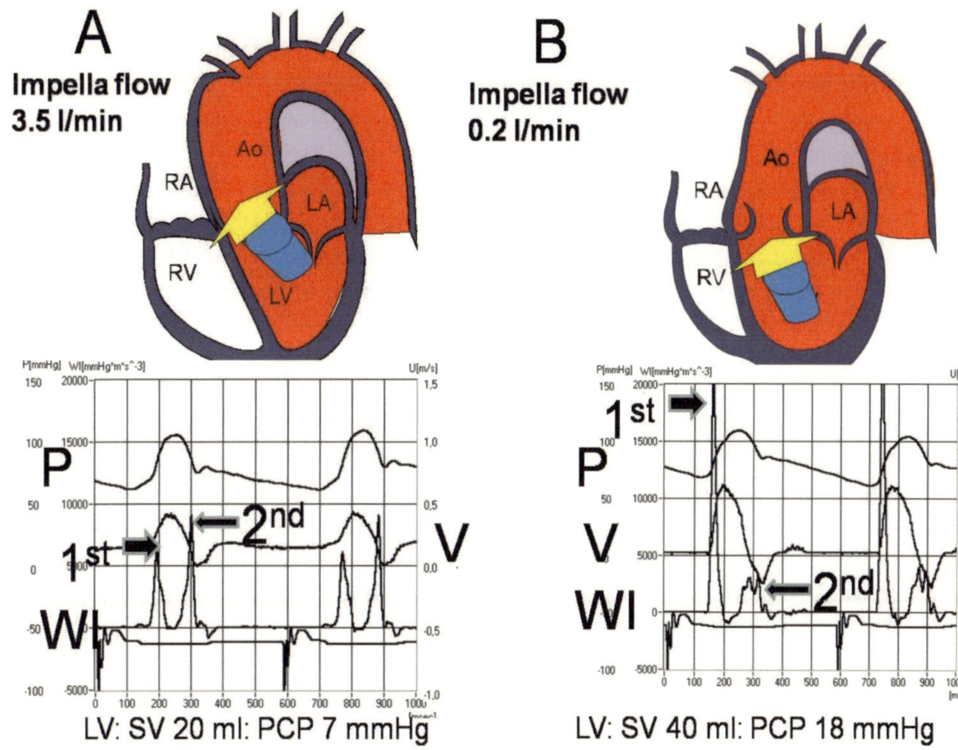

Fig. 5. The noninvasive WI 1st and 2nd peak (WI curve) assessed in the patient represented in Fig. 4, during stage A and B of Impella support. The scale is the same for A and B.
P = pressure, V = flow, SV = stroke volume, PCP = pulmonary capillary pressure

2.1.3 Effect of posture on wave intensity

WI studies in humans suffering from circulatory failure are limited to a small number of centers.[40] In 2001 we first studied 31 patients suffering from end stage DCM[41] to assess circulatory reserves by utilizing a simple tilting test moving patients from supine to upright position. When DCM patients moved from supine to upright position, the filling of the venous bed was reduced (the overdistended jugular vein was collapsed) and filling of the heart chambers was therefore also reduced. Changed preload and afterload forces influenced the mitral filling pattern of the failing myocardium as well, as recorded by pulsed Doppler. The E wave (early filling or spontaneous filling) was significantly reduced (0.7±0.22 vs 0.4±0.19 m/s, p=0.001) and the A wave (atrial kick) was unchanged (0.5±0.15

m/s vs 0.5±0.10). This alteration significantly influences in a negative manner the stroke volume (p=0.05) but not WI parameters. The 1st and 2nd peak were not significantly higher in standing than in supine position (1st 4606±2283 vs 5405±2432 and 2nd 1483±675 vs 2002 ±726 mmHg*s^3, both ns). The conclusion should be drawn that in patients suffering from chronic systolic and diastolic myocardial failure the acutely provoked hemodynamic imbalance of preload and afterload influences SV negatively, but this alteration was corrected by mechanical cooperation of the arterial conduit to keep adequate conditions in the circulation system. Therefore the wave intensity marker is helpful by providing information not only about LV systolic function but also about the mechanoelastic prosperities of the arterial system integrated with the elastic prosperities of the myocardium responsible for hemodynamic homeostasis.

2.1.4 Wave intensity as a prognostic marker

The next study at the Deutsches Herzzentrum Berlin (DHZB, German Heart Institute Berlin) was performed in a prospective manner to establish the utility of WI as a predictor of life expectancy. A cohort of 151 consecutive outpatients (age 48.7±12 years; 110 men) with end-stage DCM was prospectively studied. The follow-up period of patients was 31±8 months. End-points were death, life-saving circulatory support, and urgent transplantation.

During the follow-up 44 patients were lost; there were 15 cardiac deaths (10%), life-saving ventricular assist device implantation in 10 (6.6%) and transplantation in 19 (12.7%). The most accurate predisposing factor for events (death, assist device implantation and urgent transplantation) in ambulatory patients was low 1st peak (OR 45.6, CI 14.5-143.3, $p<0.001$) (Fig. 1). The "cut-off value" for 1st peak assessed on the basis of our study was set at the level of <4100 mmHg*s^3[42]. Less powerful predictors of the risk of deterioration were: low quotient of 1st to 2nd peak relation, left sided filling pressure (PCP), diastolic PAP and E/A mitral wave ratio (p=0.05 for all). Left ventricular ejection fraction (LVEF) and LV diameter did not show statistical significance for this purpose.

Figure 6 shows the event-free cumulative survival of ambulatory patients (n=151). This curve does not represent a pure survival curve because patients who were removed from this curve do not represent those who died, while this group includes those who were saved by transplantation or VAD implantation as well as those who died. Patients accepted in this way and regarded as "event free" represent those who were hemodynamically stable. In other words, the group of patients designated "event positive" were lost for the purposes of our study not only because of death but also because of hemodynamic instability or hemodynamic and clinical worsening; these patients could not be stabilized with medical means but required assist device implantation or urgent transplantation.

3. Discussion

The usual and until now most plausible explanation for unexpected or unpredicted worsening (transition) into "true decompensation" was based on primary systolic or diastolic myocardial failure[43,44]. In the list of probable predictors the arterial part of the circulation has been ignored as a possibly important issue where "unknown" factors could be hidden. This has led to limited interest and little evidence-based research regarding the function of the arterial system in the presence of the "failing heart"; however, the concept of a causal relation between the heart and arterial conduit failure[45] is an important topic. It should be kept in mind that the arterial tree functions as a "conductor" and plays a vital role as an active transmitter of blood to the peripheral tissue. The reactivity of the arterial system to any kind of physiological stimulation is well known from animal studies and can negatively influence study results.[46] However, patients suffering from congestive heart failure in general and especially from the advanced stages of the disease are very stable (blunted reactivity) and do not demonstrate variability of WI parameters from beat to beat. This method was validated and demonstrated good reproducibility in human beings.[47]

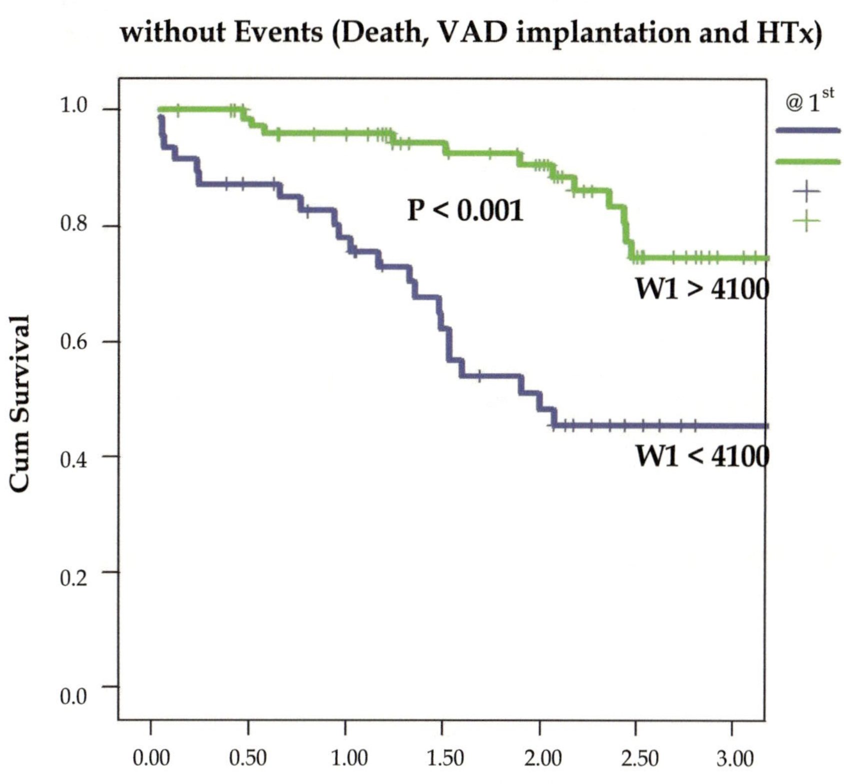

Fig. 6. "Event free" cumulative survival for ambulatory patients (n=151) divided into two groups according to the development of 1st peak WI. Survival of patients possessing WI 1st peak >4100 mmHg*s^3 (green curve); survival with the peak <4100 mmHg*s^3 (blue curve). The cut-off value of 4100 mmHg*s^3 was established empirically by studying the group of patients during "true decompensation"

3.1 Wave intensity parameters studied in carotid artery as predictors of hemodynamic deterioration

Although NWI was assessed in the carotid artery it defines the cooperation of the heart with the arterial conduit (aorta and arterial system) as a whole and not exclusively the arterial system of the heart. This is the law of "connected compartments" (vessels). Our results documented the true importance of WI assessment in defining lack of circulatory reserves, although for patients in whom heart dysfunction is present the "extracardiac" factors may play an important role in driving the patient to progressive decompensation. It has been hypothesized by others that elevated filling pressure may secondarily cause heart dysfunction but not always be the result of the loss of myocardial performance[48]. Changes in afterload are common physiological reactions of the highly sensitive arterial segment of circulation. The left ventricle "meets" directly the afterload at the end of isovolumic contraction, when the left ventricular pressure becomes equal to the aortic diastolic pressure, as stated by M. Katz. The pressure–volume relationship is strongly dependent on afterload. Increasing the afterload reduces the stroke volume of the diseased heart by increasing the pressure throughout ejection. On the contrary, decreasing the afterload reduces left ventricular pressure during ejection and increases stroke volume.[49] In other words overloading of the arterial conduit (e.g. by volume shift or sympathetic stimulation) can lead to backward LV loading above the tolerance of the diseased heart, causing smaller stroke volume. This diminution of stroke volume is difficult to assess but WI 1st peak reduction is significant. Hypervolemic episodes which lead to an afterload rise above the control ability of the diseased myocardium, do not necessarily mean simple volume overload but may represent an inter-compartment volume shift inside the circulation.[50] Newly published data supports the hypothesis that "hypervolemic episodes" are produced by volume shift in patients suffering from chronic heart failure rather than by simple external "over-supplementation." The study by Zile and coworkers[12] documented that the transition from compensation to decompensation in a group of patients suffering from chronic systolic heart failure was not bound with body weight gain and that the development of pulmonary edema was due to volume shift from one compartment to the other. Whether it was a backward or forward shift is a matter of debate. Failing interaction of the heart chambers caused by blunted vasoreflexes can cause pulmonary edema. If the right atrial filling alters in the sense that the RV increases stroke volume by only 5 ml per beat, then the LV chamber attempts to increase the stroke volume also but, if this is not possible, after 100 beats the lungs will be overloaded. On the other hand rising afterload of the LV can cause LV depression which is described as "backward" failure. The rise in afterload does not necessarily need to be connected to an arterial pressure rise but may be related to volume shift in a mechanism of reduced peripheral perfusion, as partially documented in our type B failure.

4. Conclusion

It can be hypothetically stated that heart disease is responsible for the physiological state known as heart failure but that worsening of the heart failure or recompensation should be considered dysfunction of the arterial segment of the cardiocirculation.

In general these theories support the explanation of the results of our study that cooperation between the failing heart and the arterial conduit can be an important and until recently "unknown factor" for outcome prediction in patients suffering from congestive heart failure. As we assumed, some research indicates strongly that diastolic function of the heart may be reflected in the 2nd peak[51]; this could also be interpreted as relaxation dysfunction of the LV myocardium, as we discussed in the description of "type B" pathology. In this respect WI (2nd peak) defines the diastolic function of the heart during the early phase of relaxation. However, in our study the 1st peak was found to be the most significant ($p<0.001$) prognostic factor of final hemodynamic deterioration, and this factor can be utilized in surgical decision-making for assist device implantation.

We conclude that the new ventricular-arterial coupling WI parameters assess heart-arterial conduit function. The study of arterial conduit function is promising for the prognostic assessment of patients suffering from heart failure and can help to define the optimal timing for mechanical circulatory support.

Literally the WI 1st peak can potentially be used to distinguish patients at high risk for true deterioration and death. High 2nd peak is related to severe diastolic heart failure and overvolumed arterial bed during the conversion from compensation to decompensation.

5. Acknowledgment

The authors thank Anne M. Gale for editorial assistance.

6. References

[1] Stevenson LW, Perloff JK. The limited reliability of physical signs for estimating hemodynamics in chronic heart failure. JAMA 1989;261:884-8

[2] Lee DS, Vasan RS. Novel markers for heart failure diagnosis and prognosis. *Curr Opin Cardiol.* 2005;20:201-10

[3] Stevenson WG, Stevenson LW, Middlekauff HR, Fonarow GC, Hamilton MA, Woo MA, Saxon LA, Natterson PD, Steimle A., Walden JA, Tillish JH. Improving survival for patients with advanced heart failure: A study of 737 consecutive patients. J Am Coll Cardiol 1955;26:1417-23

[4] Deng MC, De Meester JM, Smits JM, Heinecke J. Effect of receiving a heart transplant:Analysis of a national cohort entered on to a waiting list, stratified by heart failure severity. BMJ 2000;321:540-5

[5] Rieckenbacher PR, Trindade PT, Haywood GA, Vagelos RH, Schroeder JS, Willson K, Prikazsky L, Fowler, MB. Transplant candidates with severe left ventricular dysfunction managed with medical treatment: Characteristics and survival. J Am Coll Cardiol 1996;27:1192-7

[6] Lee WH, Packer M. Prognostic importance of serum sodium concentration and its modification by converting-enzyme inhibition in patients with severe chronic heart failure. Circulation, Feb 1986; 73: 257-67

[7] Abramson BL, Ando S, Notarius CF,. Rongen GA, Floras JS. Effect of atrial natriuretic peptide on muscle sympathetic activity and its reflex control in human heart failure. Circulation 1999; 99(14): 1810-15

[8] Azevedo ER, Newton GE, Floras JS, Parker D. Reducing cardiac filling pressure lowers norepinephrine spillover in patients with chronic heart failure. Circulation 2000;101(17): 2053-59

[9] Alpert JS., The effect of right ventricular dysfunction on left ventricular form and function. Chest.2001;119/6:1632-33

[10] Salvo TG, Mathier M, Semigran MJ, Dec GW. Preserved right ventricular ejection fraction predicts exercise capacity and survival in advanced heart failure. J Am Coll Cardiol 1955;25:1143-53

[11] Hassan A, Paul V. Telemonitoring in heart failure. E Heart J doi:1093/eurheart/ehr005

[12] Zile MR, Bennett TD, St. John Sutton M, Yong KC, Adamson PB., Aaron MF, Aranda JM Jr et al. Transition from chronic compensated to acute decompensated heart failure: Pathophysiological insights obtained from continuous monitoring of intracardiac pressures. Circulation, 2008; 118: 1433-41

[13] Conraads VM, Tavazzi L, Santini M, Oliva F, Gerritse B, Yu C-M. Cowie MR. Sensitivity and positive predictive value of implantable intrathoracic impedance monitoring as a predictor of heart failure hospitalizations: the SENSE-HF trial. Eur Heart J, February 28, 2011; (2011) ehr050v1

[14] Auricchio A Brugada J, Ellenbogen KA, Gold MR, Leyv F, CLEPSYDRA investigators. Assessment of a novel device-based diagnostic algorithm to monitor patient status in moderate-to-severe heart failure: rationale and design of the CLEPSYDRA study. Eur J Heart Fail 2010;12(12):1363-71

[15] Roy CS. Journal of Physiology, 1879, i, pp. 470, 496

[16] Henderson, Y. The volume curve of the ventricles of the mammalian heart, and the significance of this curve in respect to the mechanics of the heart beat and the filling of the ventricles. Am. J. Physiol. 1906;16:325

[17] Courtois M, Vered Z, Barzilai B, Ricciotti NA, Perez JE, Ludbrook PA.. The transmitral pressure-flow velocity relation effect of abrupt preload reduction. Circulation 1988;78:1459-68

[18] Guyton AC. Determination of cardiac output by equating venous return curves with cardiac response curves. Physiol Rev 1955;35:123-29

[19] Guyton AC, Hall JE. Textbook of Medical Physiology. Vascular Distensibility and Functions of the Arterial and Venous Systems. Ch 15. (12th ed.). Saunders Elsvier, 2011, p. 168

[20] GuytonAC Hall JE. Textbook of Medical Physiology. Cardiac Muscle; The Heart as a Pump and Function of the Heart Valves. Ch 9. (12th ed.). Saunders Elsvier, 2011, p. 101-113

[21] Atherton JJ, Thomson HL, Moore TD, Wright KN, Muehle GWF, Fitzpatrick E, Frenneaux MP. Diastolic ventricular interaction: A possible mechanism for abnormal vascular responses during volume unloading in heart failure. Circulation 1997;96:4273-79

[22] Kubo SH, Cody RJ. Circulatory autoregulation in chronic congestive heart failure: responses to head-up tilt in 41 patients. Am J Cardiol. 1983;52:521-28

[23] Thomson HL, Wright K, Frenneaux M. Baroreflex sensitivity in patients with vasovagal syncope. Circulation. 1997;95:395-400

[24] Thorén P. Characteristics of left ventricular receptors with non-medullated vagal afferents in cats. Circ Res. 1977;40:415-21

[25] Raphael CE, Whinnett ZI, Davies JE, Fontana M, Ferenczi EA, Manisty CH, Mayet J, Francis DP. Quantifying the paradoxical effect of higher systolic blood pressure on mortality in chronic heart failure. Heart 2009;95:56-62

[26] Pfeffer MA. Blood pressure in heart failure: a love-hate relationship. J Am Coll Cardiol 2007;49:40-42

[27] Nunez J, Nunez E, Fonarow GC, Sanchis J,. Bodi V, Bertomeu-Gonzalez V, Minana G et al. Differential prognostic effect of systolic blood pressure on mortality according to left-ventricular function in patients with acute heart failure. Eur J Heart Fail 2010; 12(1): 38-44

[28] Cohen-Solal A, Tabet JY, Logeart D, Bourgoin P, Tokmakova M, Dahan M. A non-invasively determined surrogate of cardiac power ('circulatory power') at peak exercise is a powerful prognostic factor in chronic heart failure. Eur Heart J 2002;23:806-14
[29] Noble MI. The contribution of blood momentum to left ventricular ejection in the dog. Circ Res 1968;23:663-70
[30] Spencer MP, Griess FC. Dynamics of ventricular ejection. Circ Res 1962;10: 274
[31] Parker KH., Jones CJH., Forward and backward running waves in the arteries: Analysis using the method of characteristics. J Bimech Eng 1990;112:322-26
[32] Sugawara M, Niki K, Furuhata H, Ohnishi S, Suzuki S. Relationship between pressure and diameter of the carotid artery in humans. Heart Vessels 2000;15:49-51
[33] Harada A, Okada T, Sugawara M, Niki K Development of a non-invasive real-time measurement system of wave intensity. Proceedings of IEEE Ultrasonics Symposium 2000:1517-20
[34] Katz AM. The working heart. In: Katz AM. Physiology of the Heart. Lippincott Williams and Wilkins, fifth edition 2011, p. 328
[35] Solomon S.B., Nikolic S.D., Frater R:W., Yellin E.L. Contraction-relaxation coupling: determination of the onset of diastole. Am. J. Physiol. 1999;277:H23-H27
[36] Lendrum B, Feinberg H, Boyd E, Katz LN. Rhythm effects on contractility of the beating isovolumic left ventricle. Amer J Physiol 199:1115, 1960
[37] Pace JB. Priola DV, Randall WC. Alterations in cardiac synchrony and contractility during induced pulsus alternans. Physiologist 1966;9:259
[38] Hogancam C., Kardesch M, Danforth WH, Bing RJ. Transmembrane electrical potentials in ventricular tachycardia and fibrillation. Amer Heart J 1959;57: 214
[39] Cohn KE, Sandler H, Hancock W. Mechanisms of pulsus alternans Circulation 1967; 36: 372-380.
[40] Sugawara M, Niki K, Ohte N, Okada T, Harada A. Clinical usefulness of wave intensity analysis. Med Biol Eng Comput. 2009;47:197-206.
[41] Siniawski H, Unbehaun A, Lehmkuhl H, Kapell S, Schoen F, Hetzer R. Clinical and echocardiographic features in patients with dilated cardiomyopathy: Wave intensity and diastolic abnormality analysis. Przeglad Lekarski 2002;59(8):562-67
[42] Siniawski H, Heizmann P, Lehmkuhl HB, Dandel M, Hoffmann M, Knosalla C, Pasic M, Weng Y, Stein J, Hetzer R. Echocardiographic features of early graft dysfunction after heart transplantation. 2006 World Transplant Congress, Boston, 22.-27.7.2006. American Journal of Transplantation 2006;6(Suppl 2):557
[43] Vasan SR, Levy D. Defining diastolic heart failure: A call for standardized diagnostic criteria. Circulation 2000;101:2118-21
[44] Working Group Report. How to diagnose diastolic heart failure: European Study Group on Diastolic Heart Failure. Eur Heart J. 1998;19:990-1003
[45] Petrie CJ, Robertson M, Voors AJ, Van Veldhuisen AD, Dargie HJ. Abstract 2615: A low pulse pressure predicts mortality in patients with left ventricular dysfunction post myocardial infarction, but only in those with signs and symptoms of heart failure. Circulation 2007; 116: II 579
[46] Van Vliet BN, Montaini JP. Baroreflex stabilization of the double product. Am J Physiol. 1999;277:H1679-89

[47] Niki K, Sugawara M, Chang D, Harada A, Okada T, Sakai R, Uchida K, Tanaka R, Mumford CE. A new noninvasive measurement system for wave intensity: evaluation of carotid arterial wave intensity and reproducibility. Heart Vessels 2002;17:12-2

[48] Burkhoff D, Maurer MS, Packer M. Heart failure with a normal ejection fraction: is it really a disorder of diastolic function? Circulation 2003;107:656-58

[49] Katz AM. The working heart, Ch 12. In: Katz AM Physiology of the Heart. Lippincott Williams and Wilkins, fifth edition 2011, pp. 313-42

[50] Yumino D, Redolfi S, Ruttanaumpawan P, Su MC, Smith S, Newton, GE, Mak S, Bradley TD. Nocturnal Rostral Fluid Shift: A Unifying Concept for the Pathogenesis of Obstructive and Central Sleep Apnea in Men With Heart Failure. Circulation 2010; 121; 1598-1605

[51] Jones C.J.H, Sugawara M, Kondoh Y, Uchida K, Parker K.H. Compression and expansion wavefront travel in canine ascending aortic flow: Wave intensity analysis. Heart Vessels 2002;16:91-98

2

Left Ventricular Assist Devices: Engineering Design Considerations

Marwan A. Simaan[1], George Faragallah[1], Yu Wang[1] and Eduardo Divo[2]
[1]University of Central Florida, Orlando, Florida,
[2]Daytona State College, Daytona Beach, Florida,
USA

1. Introduction

Patients with end-stage congestive heart failure awaiting heart transplantation often wait long periods of time (300 days or more on the average) before a suitable donor heart becomes available. The medical community has placed increased emphasis on the use of Left Ventricular Assist Devices or LVADs that can substitute for, or enhance, the function of the natural heart while the patient is waiting for the heart transplant (Poirier, 1997; Frazier & Myers, 1999). Essentially, a rotary LVAD is a pump that operates continuously directing blood from the left ventricle into the aorta by avoiding the aortic valve. Generally speaking, the goal of the LVAD is to assist the native heart in pumping blood through the circulatory system so as to provide the patient with as close to a normal lifestyle as possible until a donor heart becomes available or, in some cases, until the patient's heart recovers. In many situations, this means allowing the patient to return home and/or to the workforce.

The amount of blood pumped by the LVAD into the circulatory system depends on many factors, the most important of which is the rotational speed of the pump which is directly controlled by the pump motor current. The higher the speed of the pump the more blood is forced into the circulatory system. Because of this, an important engineering challenge facing the increased use of these LVADs is the development of an appropriate controller for the speed of the rotor. Such a controller, in addition to being robust and reliable, must satisfy two important criteria:

1. It must be able to adapt to the daily activities and physiological and emotional changes of the patient by regulating the pump speed in order to meet the body's requirements for cardiac output (CO) and mean arterial pressure (MAP) (Olsen, 2000; Boston et al., 2003; Schima et al., 1992; Marieb, 1994).
2. It should ensure that the rotational speed does not exceed an upper limit beyond which the pump will be attempting to draw more blood from the ventricle than available. The occurrence of this phenomenon, known as suction, for a brief period of time may cause collapse of the ventricle resulting in damage to the heart muscle (Yuhki et al. 1999; Vollkron et al., 2006; Ferreira et al., 2006). Suction, therefore, must be detected quickly and the pump speed reduced before any damage to the heart muscle occurs.

The eventual goal of an LVAD speed controller is therefore to meet the above two requirements so that an LVAD recipient patient could potentially leave the hospital and return home to a safe and normal lifestyle. Given that the pump is continuously interacting with the left ventricle and circulatory system, the development of a speed controller must therefore be done using engineering tools that require a mathematical model of the entire system. The model must be simple enough to be tractable and yet it must be comprehensive enough to capture the essential relationships between the hemodynamic variables and their interactions with the LVAD without the ambiguity of including unnecessary state variables. In this chapter, we discuss the development of such a model. We will first review an autonomous 5th order model of the cardiovascular system, which emphasizes the pressure-volume relationship of the left ventricle. We then present a 1st order model of a rotary LVAD along with its inflow and outflow cannulae and with the pump motor current as its control variable. This model is a variation from the model described in (Simaan et al.; 2009; Simaan, 2009) where the rotational speed was assumed to be the control variable. In reality, the only way the speed can be varied is by varying the pump motor current through a very complex relationship. We account for the phenomenon of suction by adding a nonlinear resistance to the inflow cannula model which becomes active when the left ventricular pressure drops below a certain threshold. Finally, we combine these two models into a 6th order time varying nonlinear model with the pump motor current being the only control variable. The time variations in this model are due to the cyclical nature of the ventricle elastance and its changes as a function of time within one cardiac cycle. The nonlinearities are due to the mitral and aortic valves in the cardiovascular model and the suction resistance in the LVAD model. The binary state of each of these valves yields four consecutive phases within one cardiac cycle during which the ventricle contracts, ejects, relaxes and then fills depending on which valve is open and which is closed. As a result, the mathematical description of the entire model changes as the ventricle crosses from one phase to the next. We will conclude this chapter by outlining some of the challenges in the development of both a feedback speed controller and a suction detection algorithm that need to be overcome before the ultimate goal of the LVAD becomes a reality as well as a discussion of a new Computational Fluid Dynamics (CFD) model of the aortic arch and a Lagrangian particle-tracking model to predict the path of thrombi of different sizes and initial locations traveling across the cardiovascular system. Preliminary results described in this chapter indicate that alignment of the LVAD outflow cannula at different angles of incidence as well as implantation of aortic-to-innominate bypass or aortic-to-left-carotid bypass significantly alters thrombo-embolism rates.

2. The left ventricle circulatory system model

The heart is a very complex system that is very difficult to model mathematically. In research that involves engineering considerations, the development of a mathematical model for the heart is crucial. The model should be complex enough to reproduce the performance of the heart, yet it should be also simple for the computation purposes. For these reasons, we will start, in this section, with a basic model that will be used in the development of feedback controller and suction detection algorithms. Later in the chapter, we will introduce a more complex multi degree-of-freedom (DOF) model that is used in the computational fluid dynamics analysis for prevention of trombo-embolism events.

The basis model assumes that the right ventricle and pulmonary circulation are healthy and normal and as a result their effect on the LVAD can be neglected. A 5th order lumped parameter electric circuit model which can reproduce the left ventricle hemodynamics of the heart (Simaan et al., 2009) is shown in Figure 1. In this model, the behavior of the left

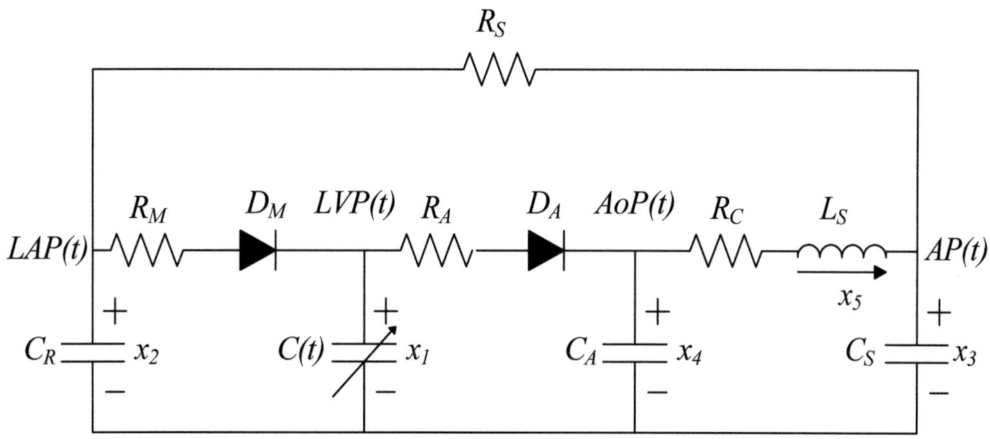

Fig. 1. Cardiovascular electric circuit model

ventricle is modeled by means of a time varying capacitance (or compliance) C(t), which is the reciprocal of the ventricle's elastance function E(t). The elastance represents the contractual state of the left ventricle. It relates to the ventricle's pressure and volume (Suga and Sagawa, 1974) according to the expression:

$$E(t) = \frac{LVP(t)}{LVV(t) - V_0} \tag{1}$$

where LVP(t) is the left ventricular pressure, LVV(t) is the left ventricular volume, and V_0 is a reference volume, which corresponds to the theoretical volume in the ventricle at zero pressure. The elastance function E(t) can be approximated mathematically. In our work we use the expression:

$$E_H(t) = (E_{max} - E_{min})E_n(t_n) + E_{min} \tag{2}$$

where $E_H(t)$ represents the elastance of a healthy heart, $E_n(t_n)$ is the normalized elastance (also called "double hill" function) represented by the expression (Stergiopoulos et al., 1996a):

$$E_n(t_n) = 1.55 \cdot \left[\frac{\left(\frac{t_n}{0.7}\right)^{1.9}}{1 + \left(\frac{t_n}{0.7}\right)^{1.9}} \right] \cdot \left[\frac{1}{1 + \left(\frac{t_n}{1.17}\right)^{21.9}} \right] \tag{3}$$

In the above expression, $E_n(t_n)$ is the normalized elastance, $t_n = t/T_{max}$, $T_{max} = 0.2 + 0.15t_c$ and t_c is the cardiac cycle interval, i.e., $t_c = 60/HR$, where HR is the heart-rate. Notice that $E_H(t)$ is a re-scaled version of $E_n(t_n)$ and the constants E_{max} and E_{min} are related to the end-systolic pressure volume relationship (ESPVR) and the end-diastolic pressure volume relationship (EDPVR) respectively. Figure 2 shows a plot of $E_H(t)$ for a healthy heart with E_{max}= 2 mmHg/ml and E_{min}=0.06 mmHg/ml, and a heart-rate of 60 beats per minute (bpm). For a heart with cardiovascular disease, the elastance expression used in our model is modified according to $E(t)=\delta E_H(t)$. That is, the elastance E(t) is scaled version of $E_H(t)$ with a factor $0<\delta\leq 1$ where $\delta=1$ represents a healthy heart and smaller values of δ are used to represent cardiovascular disease. The more severe the disease is, the smaller the value of δ. Also in the model preload and pulmonary circulations are represented by the capacitance C_R; the aortic compliance is represented by the capacitance C_A, and afterload is represented by the four-element Windkessel model (Stergiopoulos et al., 1996b) comprising R_C, L_S, C_S and R_S. Preload, or venous blood returning to the heart, is closely related to the cardiac output (CO) produced by the heart for a given level of contractility. Afterload can be described as the pressure that the left ventricle has to generate in order to eject blood. It refers to the vascular resistance that the heart sees as it pumps blood. The mitral and aortic valves are represented by two non-ideal diodes consisting of a resistance R_M and ideal diode D_M for the mitral valve, and resistance R_A and ideal diode D_A for the aortic valve. In this representation, we have kept the number of model parameters at a minimum while maintaining enough complexity in the model so that it can reproduce the hemodynamics of the left ventricle. Table 1 lists the various system parameters and their typical associated values (Yu et al. 1998).

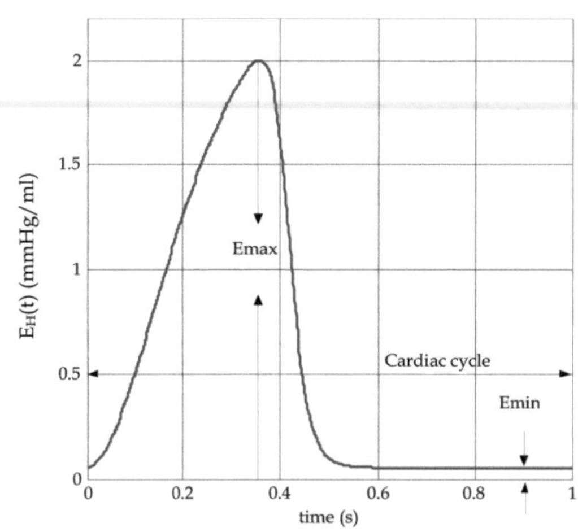

Fig. 2. Elastance function E(t)=1/C(t) of a healthy heart. (Cardiac Cycle =60/HR)

Obviously the circuit model in Figure 1 is time-varying because of the time dependence in C(t) and nonlinear because of the two diodes. Since each diode has two states: open-circuit (o/c) and short-circuit (s/c), four different circuits representing the four different phases of the ventricular functions can therefore be modeled. When the mitral valve is open and aortic valve is closed (i.e. D_M is s/c and D_A is o/c) the circuit in Figure 1 represents the phase when the left ventricle is filling. When the mitral valve is closed and the aortic valve is open (i.e. D_M is o/c and D_A is s/c) the circuit represents the phase when the ventricle is ejecting. When both the mitral and aortic valves are closed (i.e. D_M and D_A are o/c), which occurs twice, the circuit represents the two phases when the ventricle is undergoing isovolumic contraction and relaxation. Finally, the phase when both the mitral and aortic valves are open (i.e. both diodes are s/c) is clearly not feasible. The three different phases of operation of the left ventricle within the cardiac cycle are summarized in Table 2. Every phase is therefore modeled by a different equivalent circuit and hence a different set of linear time-varying differential equations. Instead of writing three different sets of differential equations, by appropriately modeling the diodes as nonlinear elements, it is possible to write only one set of equations, which describes the behavior of the entire model for all three phases. Selecting the state variables as the hemodynamic variables listed in Table 3 (and shown on the circuit in Figure 1), and using basic circuit analysis techniques (Dorf & Svoboda, 2006) such as Kirchhoff's Voltage and Current Laws (KVL and KCL) we can derive the state equations for the cardiovascular circuit model shown in Figure 1 as follows:

Parameters	Value	Physiological Meaning
Resistances (mmHg · s/ml)		
R_S	1.0000	Systemic Vascular Resistance (SVR)
R_M	0.0050	Mitral Valve Resistance
R_A	0.0010	Aortic Valve Resistance
R_C	0.0398	Characteristic Resistance
Compliances (ml/mmHg)		
C(t)	Time-varying	Left Ventricular Compliance
C_R	4.4000	Left Atrial Compliance
C_S	1.3300	Systemic Compliance
C_A	0.0800	Aortic Compliance
Inertances (mmHg · s^2/ml)		
L_S	0.0005	Inertance of blood in Aorta
Valves		
D_M		Mitral Valve
D_A		Aortic Valve

Table 1. Model parameters

Modes	Valves		Phases
	Mitral	Aortic	
1	Closed	Closed	Isovolumic Relaxation
2	Open	Closed	Filling
1	Closed	Closed	Isovolumic Contraction
3	Closed	Open	Ejection
-	Open	Open	Not feasible

Table 2. Ventricular phases within one cardiac cycle

Variables	Name	Physiological Meaning (units)
$x_1(t)$	LVP(t)	Left Ventricular Pressure (mmHg)
$x_2(t)$	LAP(t)	Left Atrial Pressure (mmHg)
$x_3(t)$	AP(t)	Arterial Pressure (mmHg)
$x_4(t)$	AoP(t)	Aortic Pressure (mmHg)
$x_5(t)$	$Q_T(t)$	Total flow (ml/s)

Table 3. State variables in the left ventricle circulatory model

$$\begin{bmatrix}\dot{x}_1\\ \dot{x}_2\\ \dot{x}_3\\ \dot{x}_4\\ \dot{x}_5\end{bmatrix}=\begin{bmatrix}\frac{-\dot{C}(t)}{C(t)} & 0 & 0 & 0 & 0\\ 0 & \frac{-1}{R_S C_R} & \frac{1}{R_S C_R} & 0 & 0\\ 0 & \frac{1}{R_S C_S} & \frac{-1}{R_S C_S} & 0 & \frac{1}{C_S}\\ 0 & 0 & 0 & 0 & \frac{-1}{C_A}\\ 0 & 0 & \frac{-1}{L_S} & \frac{1}{L_S} & \frac{-R_C}{L_S}\end{bmatrix}\begin{bmatrix}x_1\\ x_2\\ x_3\\ x_4\\ x_5\end{bmatrix}+\begin{bmatrix}\frac{1}{C(t)} & \frac{-1}{C(t)}\\ \frac{-1}{C_R} & 0\\ 0 & 0\\ 0 & \frac{1}{C_A}\\ 0 & 0\end{bmatrix}\begin{bmatrix}\frac{1}{R_M} r(x_2-x_1)\\ \frac{1}{R_A} r(x_1-x_4)\end{bmatrix} \quad (4)$$

In the above expression $r(\xi)$ represents the ramp function:

$$r(\xi)=\begin{cases}\xi & \text{if} \quad \xi \geq 0\\ 0 & \text{if} \quad \xi < 0\end{cases} \quad (5)$$

We note that the model described above is an autonomous system that does not have an input variable. Validation of this system can be found in (Simaan et al., 2009).

3. The LVAD pump motor current model

The LVAD considered in this paper is a rotary mechanical pump connected with two cannulae between the left ventricle and the aorta. The LVAD pumps blood continuously from the left ventricle into the aorta. The pressure difference between the left ventricle and the aorta is characterized by the following relationship:

$$LVP(t) - AoP(t) = R_i Q + L_i \frac{dQ}{dt} + R_o Q + L_o \frac{dQ}{dt} + R_p Q + L_p \frac{dQ}{dt} - H_p + R_{su} Q \quad (6)$$

In the above expression, H_p is the pressure (head) gain across the pump and Q is the blood flow rate through the pump. The parameters, R_i, R_o, and R_p represent the flow resistances and L_i, L_o, and L_p represent the flow inertances of the cannulae and pump respectively. Values for these parameters are shown in Table 4.

Parameters	Value	Physiological Meaning
Cannulae Resistances ($mmHg \cdot s/ml$)		
R_i	0.0677	Inlet Cannula Resistance
R_p	0.17070	Pump Resistance
R_o	0.0677	Outflow Cannula Resistance
Cannulae Inertances ($mmHg \cdot s^2/ml$)		
L_i	0.0127	Inlet Cannula Inertance
L_p	0.02177	Pump Inertance
L_o	0.0127	Outflow Cannula Inertance

Table 4. Parameter values in LVAD model

The nonlinear time-varying resistance R_{su} in (6) has the form:

$$R_{su} = \begin{cases} 0 & \text{if} \quad LVP(t) > \bar{x}_1 \\ \alpha(LVP(t)-\bar{x}_1) & \text{if} \quad LVP(t) \le \bar{x}_1 \end{cases} \tag{7}$$

It is included in the model to characterize the phenomenon of suction. Clearly, R_{su} is zero when the pump is operating normally and is activated when LVP(t) (x_1) becomes less than a predetermined small threshold $\bar{x}_1$, a condition that represents suction. The value of R_{su} when suction occurs increases linearly as a function of the difference between LVP(t) and $\bar{x}_1$. The parameter α is a cannula dependent scaling factor. The values used for the suction parameters are α = -3.5 s/ml and $\bar{x}_1$=1 mmHg.
The pressure gain across the pump H_p is modeled using the direct relation between the electric power supplied to the pump motor P_e and the hydrodynamic power generated by the pump P_p scaled by the pump efficiency η as $P_p=\eta P_e$. Furthermore, the electric power may be written in terms of the supplied voltage V and the supplied current i(t) to the pump motor as $P_e=Vi(t)$, while the hydrodynamic power may be written in terms of the pump head or pressure gain H_p and the pump flow Q as $P_p=\rho g H_p Q$, (Faragallah et al, 2011) where ρ is the density of the reference fluid and g is the acceleration of gravity (ρ_{Hg}=13,600 kg/m^3, g=9.8 m/s^2). Combining these expressions yields:

$$H_p = \frac{\eta V}{\rho g} \cdot \frac{i(t)}{Q} \tag{8}$$

or,

$$H_p = \gamma \frac{i(t)}{Q} \tag{9}$$

where $\gamma = \eta V/\rho g$. For a typical LVAD, after applying the appropriate conversion factors and assuming a pump motor supplied voltage V=12 volts as well as a pump efficiency of 100% (assuming that most losses are accounted for by the pressure losses induced by R_p and L_p), the constant γ can be computed to be γ = 89,944 mmHg$\cdot$ml/s$\cdot$amp.
Substituting (9) in (6) we obtain the nonlinear state equation governing the behavior of the LVAD as:

$$LVP(t) - AoP(t) = R^{*}Q + L^{*}\frac{dQ}{dt} - \gamma \frac{i(t)}{Q} \tag{10}$$

where $R^*=R_i+R_o+R_p+R_{su}$ and $L^*=L_i+L_o+L_p$. Note that it is important to validate the numerical solution when expression (10) is used by ensuring that the system does not allow for operation at zero pump flow Q(t) at any point during the cardiac cycle since equation (10) exhibits its nonlinearity with the pump flow Q(t) in the denominator. Using the relation between the pump pressure H_p and the pump speed $\omega(t)$ (Simaan et al., 2009)) $H_p=\beta\omega^2(t)$, an expression for the pump speed in terms of the pump motor current can be derived as follows:

$$\omega(t) = \sqrt{\frac{\gamma i(t)}{\beta Q(t)}} \tag{11}$$

where $\beta=9.9025 \cdot 10^{-7}$ mmHg/(rpm)^2. Note that it is now clear how the heart hemodynamics through Q(t) influence directly, in a highly nonlinear manner, the pump speed $\omega(t)$.

4. The combined model with pump motor current as the control variable

The addition of the LVAD to the left ventricle model in (4) will yield the 6th order system shown in Figure 3 and described by the differential equations:

$$\begin{bmatrix} \dot{x}_1 \\ \dot{x}_2 \\ \dot{x}_3 \\ \dot{x}_4 \\ \dot{x}_5 \\ \dot{x}_6 \end{bmatrix} = \begin{bmatrix} \frac{-\dot{C}(t)}{C(t)} & 0 & 0 & 0 & 0 & \frac{-1}{C(t)} \\ 0 & \frac{-1}{R_S C_R} & \frac{1}{R_S C_R} & 0 & 0 & 0 \\ 0 & \frac{1}{R_S C_S} & \frac{-1}{R_S C_S} & 0 & \frac{1}{C_S} & 0 \\ 0 & 0 & 0 & 0 & \frac{-1}{C_A} & \frac{1}{C_A} \\ 0 & 0 & \frac{-1}{L_S} & \frac{1}{L_S} & \frac{-R_C}{L_S} & 0 \\ \frac{1}{L^*} & 0 & 0 & \frac{-1}{L^*} & 0 & \frac{-R^*}{L^*} \end{bmatrix} \begin{bmatrix} x_1 \\ x_2 \\ x_3 \\ x_4 \\ x_5 \\ x_6 \end{bmatrix} + \begin{bmatrix} \frac{1}{C(t)} & \frac{-1}{C(t)} \\ \frac{-1}{C_R} & 0 \\ 0 & 0 \\ 0 & \frac{1}{C_A} \\ 0 & 0 \\ 0 & 0 \end{bmatrix} \begin{bmatrix} \frac{1}{R_M} r(x_2 - x_1) \\ \frac{1}{R_A} r(x_1 - x_4) \end{bmatrix} + \begin{bmatrix} 0 \\ 0 \\ 0 \\ 0 \\ 0 \\ \frac{\gamma}{L^* x_6} \end{bmatrix} i(t) \quad (12)$$

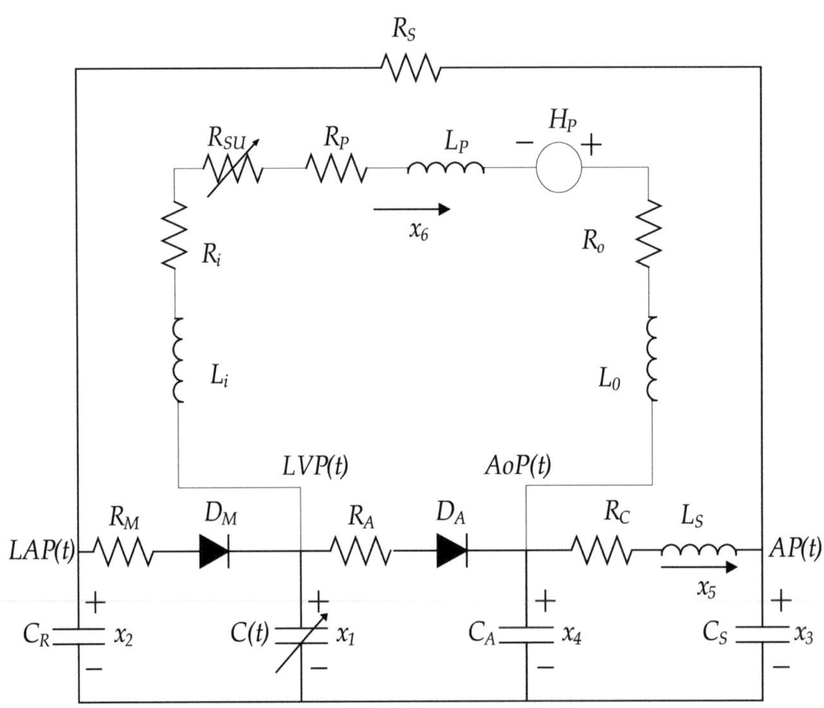

Fig. 3. Combined cardiovascular and LVAD model

Note that the additional state variable $x_6(t)=Q(t)$ represents the blood flow through the pump. Eight other passive variables: R_i, R_p, R_o, R_{su}, L_i, L_p, L_o (see Table 4) and a parameter γ have also been added. The combined model (12) is now a forced system where the control variable is the supplied current to the pump motor i(t).
Note that one of the state variables, specifically $x_6(t)$, appears in the denominator of the right-hand side of the system in (12). Therefore, special care must be taken in the numerical solution of the system as the non-linearity can significantly affect the stability of the solution algorithm. In this case, a simple time-lagging combined with a sub-level iteration scheme was devised to control the stability of the numerical solution process.

5. Considerations in the development of a feedback controller

Clearly the model derived above allows for the LVAD to be controlled by its pump motor i(t) instead of its pump speed $\omega(t)$. In this model i(t) must be adjusted to meet the patient needs for cardiac output while at the same time keeping the speed in the safe region to avoid suction. Since until very recently, most LVAD models have used the pump speed as the control variable, it is important at this stage to validate the model by examining how the pump speed is affected when using the pump motor current i(t) as the control variable.

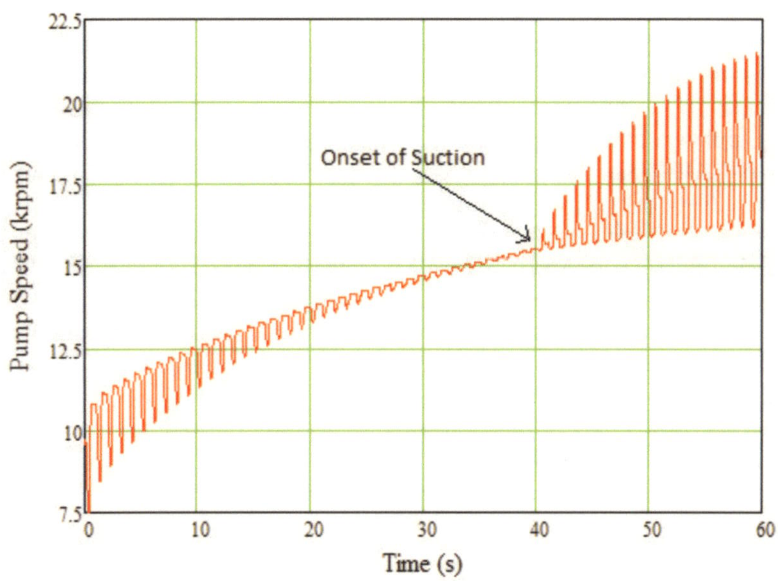

Fig. 4. Pump speed signal as a function of time derived from our model when the pump motor current is increased linearly

Figure 4 shows a plot of the pump speed when the model, with a heart rate HR=60 bpm, is excited with a linearly increasing pump current starting at i(0)=0.1 amp and increasing with a slope m=0.01 amp/s. There are several important observations that can be made from this figure. First, note that the resulting pump speed $\omega(t)$ does not also increase linearly. Instead, it increases nonlinearly with a decreasing rate of increase. Second, the pump speed has a superposed oscillatory component that has the same pulsatility as HR. This is a very interesting and an extremely important new phenomenon that has recently been observed in in-vivo data obtained through clinical studies of intensive care patients implanted with LVADs (Mason et al. 2008). This is the first time that such a phenomenon has been reproduced from a combined cardiovascular and LVAD model and represents a breakthrough in accurately modeling this complex bio-mechanical system.

A third observation that can be made from Figure 4 is that the amplitude of the oscillatory component in the pump speed signal $\omega(t)$ seems to decrease in time up to a point when a breakdown occurs and the amplitude exhibits a sudden increase when the pump current is increased beyond this point. In Figure 4 this breakdown occurs at t=40 s which corresponds to a pump speed of 15,500 rpm. Clearly this value of pump speed corresponds to the onset of suction as will be discussed in the next section.

6. Considerations in the development of suction detection algorithm

An important constraint that should be taken into consideration in designing any LVAD controller is to ensure that the pump is rotated at a speed below a threshold beyond which the pump will attempt to draw more blood from the left ventricle than available causing a phenomenon called ventricular suction. This phenomenon, which could cause collapse of the ventricle, is dangerous and needs to be detected and corrected immediately by decreasing the pump motor current, hence lowering the pump speed below the suction threshold.

Several approaches have been used to detect suction. Among these are ones that extract features from the pump flow signal. This signal is one of very few signals that can be easily measured. These approaches use powerful pattern recognition algorithms to classify the signal into being in or out of suction. These classifiers vary from simple threshold comparisons (Oshikawa et al., 2000) to more complex techniques such as Classification and Regression Tree (CART) (Karantonis et al., 2006), Discriminant Analysis (DA) (Ferreira et al., 2006), and Neural Networks (NN) (Karantonis et al., 2008).

In this chapter, we describe a new suction detection and classification algorithm based on the Lagrangian Support Vector Machine (LSVM) method in pattern recognition (Wang et al., 2011). The LSVM is a modified version of the standard Support Vector Machine (SVM) and is characterized by high accuracy, stable performance, and fast learning speed. Several real-time applications of the SVM method in different fields have been reported in the literature (Sitaram et al., 2011; Gabran et al., 2009).

Figure 5 shows the flow chart of the proposed algorithm. The feature extraction module calculates several indices from the processed pump flow. These indices then allow a determination of the pump status as one of three states separated by two threshold values on the quantity:

$$\Delta P = MLVP\text{-}MPIP$$

where MLVP is the Minimum Left Ventricular Pressure and MPIP is the Minimum Pump Inlet Pressure. The low threshold ΔP_{NS} is the No Suction threshold and the high threshold ΔP_S is the Suction threshold. The three states of the pump status are:

1. *No Suction (NS):* This corresponds to the normal operating condition of the pump. This state is characterized by $\Delta P \leq \Delta P_{NS}$. In this case, the pump flow signal is periodic with a large sinusoidal component.
2. *Approaching Suction (AS):* In this case, $\Delta P_{NS} < \Delta P \leq \Delta P_S$ which means MPIP decreases much faster than MLVP causing ΔP to increase. The pump flow signal becomes less pulsatile compared to the No Suction case.

3. *Suction (S):* In this case $\Delta P > \Delta P_S$. During this event, the inlet cannula is evidently obstructed, MPIP exhibits very large negative spikes, and MLVP is slightly less than zero. The pump flow signal exhibits complex non-periodic behavior with a sudden large drop in the slope of the envelope of the minimum pump flow signal.

Several indices based on time domain, frequency domain, and time-frequency domain can be extracted from the pump flow signal $x_6(t)$ to use in the classifier (Ferreira et al. 2006). In this chapter we describe three possible time-domain indices, SI_1, SI_2 and SI_3, two frequency-domain indices SI_4 and SI_5, and one time-frequency domain index SI_6 for a total of six possible indices that are used by the LSVM classifier.

The first time domain index SI_1 is defined as follows (Vollkron, et al. 2004):

$$SI_1 = \frac{2 \times \mathrm{mean}(x_6(t)) - [\max(x_6(t)) + \min(x_6(t))]}{\max(x_6(t)) - \min(x_6(t))} \tag{13}$$

where mean (z(t)), max(z(t) and min(z(t)) denote the mean, maximum and minimum values of signal z(t) respectively. When suction is absent, the mean pump flow value is approximately half of the sum of the maximum and minimum values of pump flow, which shifts slightly towards minimum pump flow while approaching suction. When suction occurs, the mean pump flow value is close to the maximum pump flow value. Hence, SI_1 increases dramatically.

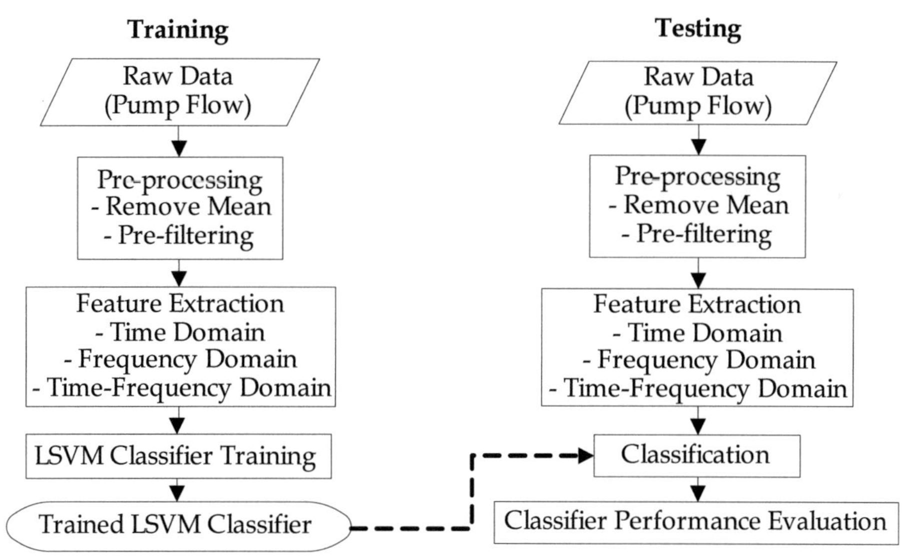

Fig. 5. Flow chart of the proposed suction detection algorithm

The other two indices SI_2 and SI_3 are calculated in terms of the derivative of the pump flow signal $x_6(t)$ as follows:

$$SI_2 = \frac{\max\left[\frac{dx_6(t)}{dt}\right]}{\max(x_6(t)) - \min(x_6(t))} \text{ and } SI_3 = \frac{\min\left[\frac{dx_6(t)}{dt}\right]}{\max(x_6(t)) - \min(x_6(t))} \tag{14}$$

Obviously SI_2 increases during suction, whereas SI_3 decreases at the beginning of suction. The frequency-domain indices SI_4 and SI_5 are calculated as follows (Ferreira et al., 2006):

$$SI_4 = \frac{\int_{\omega_1}^{\omega_2} |Q_p(\omega)| d\omega}{\int_{\omega_2}^{\infty} |Q_p(\omega)| d\omega} \text{ and } SI_5 = \frac{\int_{0}^{\omega_1} |Q_p(\omega)| d\omega}{\int_{\omega_1}^{\omega_2} |Q_p(\omega)| d\omega} \quad (15)$$

where $Q_P(\omega)$ is the Fourier transform of the pump flow signal $x_6(t)$ and ω_0 is the fundamental frequency in this signal, $\omega_1=\omega_0-\omega_c$ and $\omega_2=\omega_0+\omega_c$, where ω_c is a threshold (in radians) that defines an interval centered at ω_0. The index SI_4 is a measure of the ratio of the signal's total energy in the fundamental component frequency band to the total energy in the harmonic component frequency band and SI_5 is a measure of the ratio of the subharmonic energy to the fundamental energy. When approaching suction, SI_4 starts to decrease and SI_5 starts to increase. When suction starts, SI_4 decreases and SI_5 increases abruptly. This is due to the shift of energy from the fundamental band to both the harmonic and subharmonic bands, indicating that suction is taking place.
Finally the time-frequency-domain index SI_6 is defined as the standard deviation of instantaneous mean frequency of the pump flow signal expressed as (Ferreira et al., 2006):

$$SI_6 = \sqrt{\mathrm{var}(\langle \omega \rangle_t^{sp})} \quad (16)$$

where the instantaneous frequency is defined as the average frequency at a given time (Cohen, 1995) and expressed as:

$$\langle \omega \rangle_t^{sp} = \frac{\int \omega P_{sp}(\omega,t) d\omega}{\int P_{sp}(\omega,t) d\omega} \quad (17)$$

where $P_{SP}(\omega,t)$ is the squared magnitude of the short-time Fourier transform (STFT). The value of SI_6 is small when suction is not occurring and increases slightly when suction is approaching, and it increases abruptly when suction starts.
We will now illustrate the performance of the LSVM classifier. Figure 6(a) shows a pump flow signal of an LVAD in vivo experiment used in (Ferreira et al., 2006). The six suction indices derived from this signal are also plotted on the same figure. The changes in these indices as the pump flow signal transitions from NS to AS then to S are clearly evident in Figure 6(b)-(g). These indices are used as inputs to the LSVM classifier. The classifier is trained on a randomly selected set of 50% of the data and then tested on the remaining 50% of the data. The two thresholds on ΔP used in the classifier, as mentioned earlier, where chosen as ΔP_{NS}=10 mmHg and ΔP_S=35 mmHg. Due to the random selection of data samples, the classification is repeated 100 times. The average classification results of the proposed algorithm over 100 runs on the test set are shown in Table 5.

	NS	AS	S	Total
NS	703.14	53.36	0.5	757
AS	37.33	598.24	5.43	641
S	0.09	5.31	94.6	100

Table 5. Classification results of the LSVM Classifier (actual classes are in rows, predicted classes are in columns)

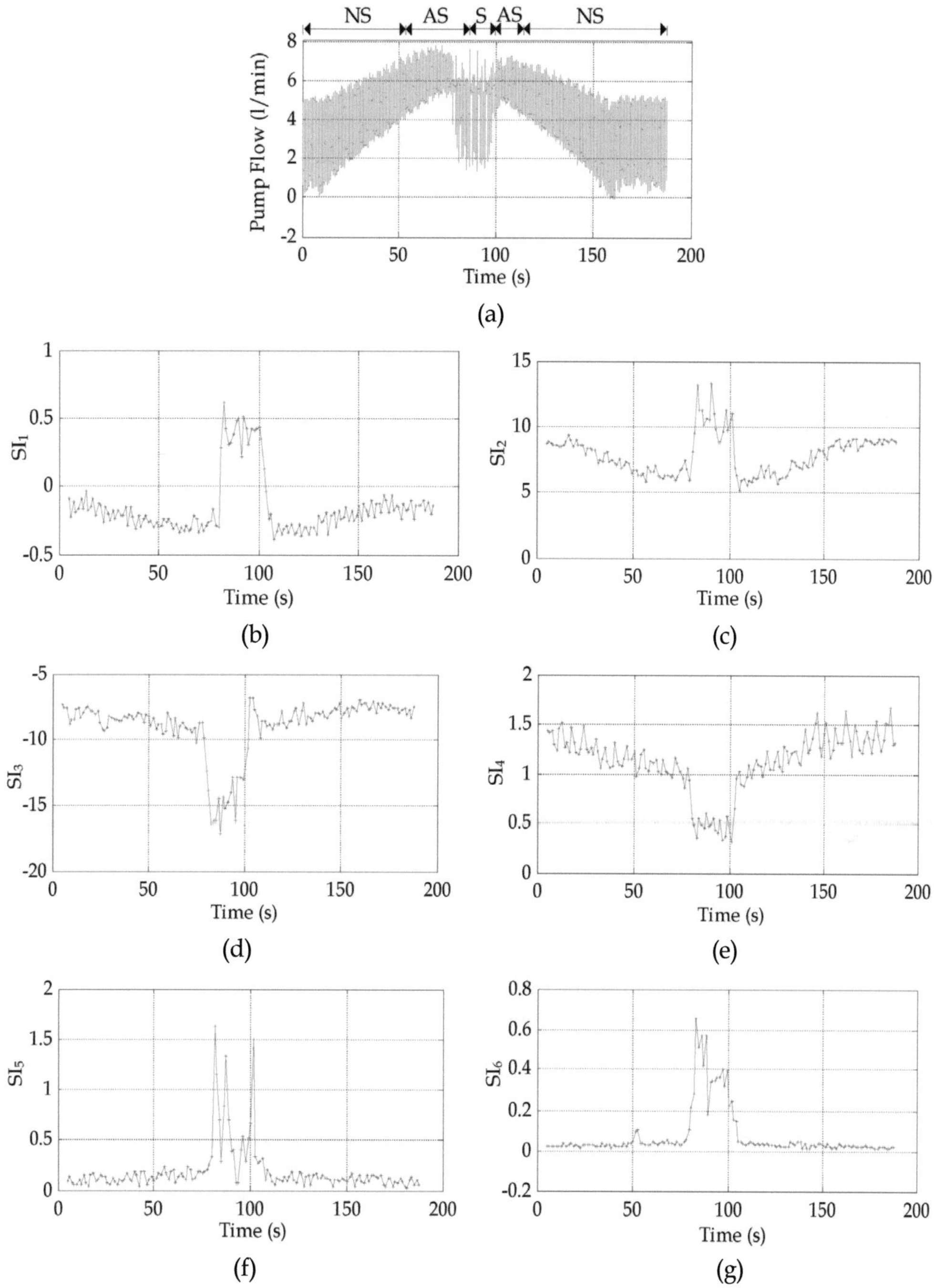

Fig. 6. Suction indices extracted from the pump flow. (a) Pump Flow. (b) SI_1. (c) SI_2. (d) SI_3. (e) SI_4. (f) SI_5. (g) SI_6

For NS, on average there are 53.36 samples misclassified as AS (7.05%) and only 0.5 samples are misclassified as S (0.06%). For AS, on average 37.33 samples are misclassified as NS

(5.82%) and only 5.43 samples are incorrectly identified as S (0.85%). For S, on average the erroneous number of samples misclassified as NS and AS are as low as 0.09 (0.09%) and 5.31 (5.31%), respectively.

7. Considerations in adjustment of angle of incidence in LVAD implantation

Like suction, stroke is another crucial complication that may result due to LVAD therapy. The incidence of such thrombo-embolic cerebral events is reduced by anticoagulation management and improved LVAD design. Still, the incidence of such events is relatively high accounting for about 19% of patients and a mortality rate of 65% (Davies et al., 2008, Russo et al., 2009, Thoennissen et al., 2006, and Schmid et al., 1998). It may be hypothesized that cerebral thrombo-embolism may be reduced by adjusting the placement and angle of incidence of the LVAD outflow cannula as well as by the implantation of an aortic-to-innominate artery bypass or an aortic-to-left-carotid artery bypass. In this section, results are presented of a numerical study conducted based on a multi-scale model where the electric circuit model of the cardiovascular/LVAD circulation as the one previously discussed is used to impose the transient fluid flow boundary conditions at the aortic arch circulation by coupling it with a Computational Fluid Dynamics (CFD) model and a Lagrangian particle-tracking model to predict the path of thrombi of different sizes and initial locations traveling across the cardiovascular system.

In order to properly account for the unsteady nature of the flow field generated by the cardiac ejection in an Aortic Arch with an implanted LVAD a closed-loop external vascular model is necessary. Such external model is coupled to the CFD model to dictate the flow field boundary conditions at the outlets of the CFD model and thus, control the flow splits through the different branches that stem out of the aortic arch throughout the cardiac cycle. To this end, a Multi-DOF (degrees of freedom) electric circuit model representing the different flow and pressure values at the different elements of the external cardiovascular model was constructed as seen in Figure 7.

We utilize the CFD code, STARCCM+, in which a Lagrangian particle-tracking model is coupled to the fluid flow solver to predict particle trajectories. In this study, we then explore the possibility of finding an optimal configuration of the LVAD conduit angle and anastomosis location (that is both distance from the innominate and polar angle in the coronal plane of the ascending aorta), and we seek to establish the benefits of the ligation of the innominate artery and placement of an aortic-to-innominate artery bypass graft or the ligation of the left carotid artery and placement of an aortic-to-left-carotid artery bypass graft.

As a preliminary approach to solve this problem, the LVAD conduit flow is assumed to be steady (non-pulsatile), with negligible pulsatile flow originating from the aortic root. Although not always the case, steady or near steady flow characterizes the flow regime in many patient with LVAD support (Shahcheraghi et al., 2002; Tokuda et al., 2008; and Drummond et al., 2008). Continuous-flow LVADs have predominantly become the device of choice. Consequently, the focus of this study is to investigate steady flow conditions and therefore, steady flow splits are imposed as boundary conditions at the outlet branches of the aortic arch rather than coupling this with the Multi-DOF electric circuit model in Figure 7. Future studies will be conducted taking into account the unsteady behavior of the flow field and the interaction with the external cardiovascular circuit.

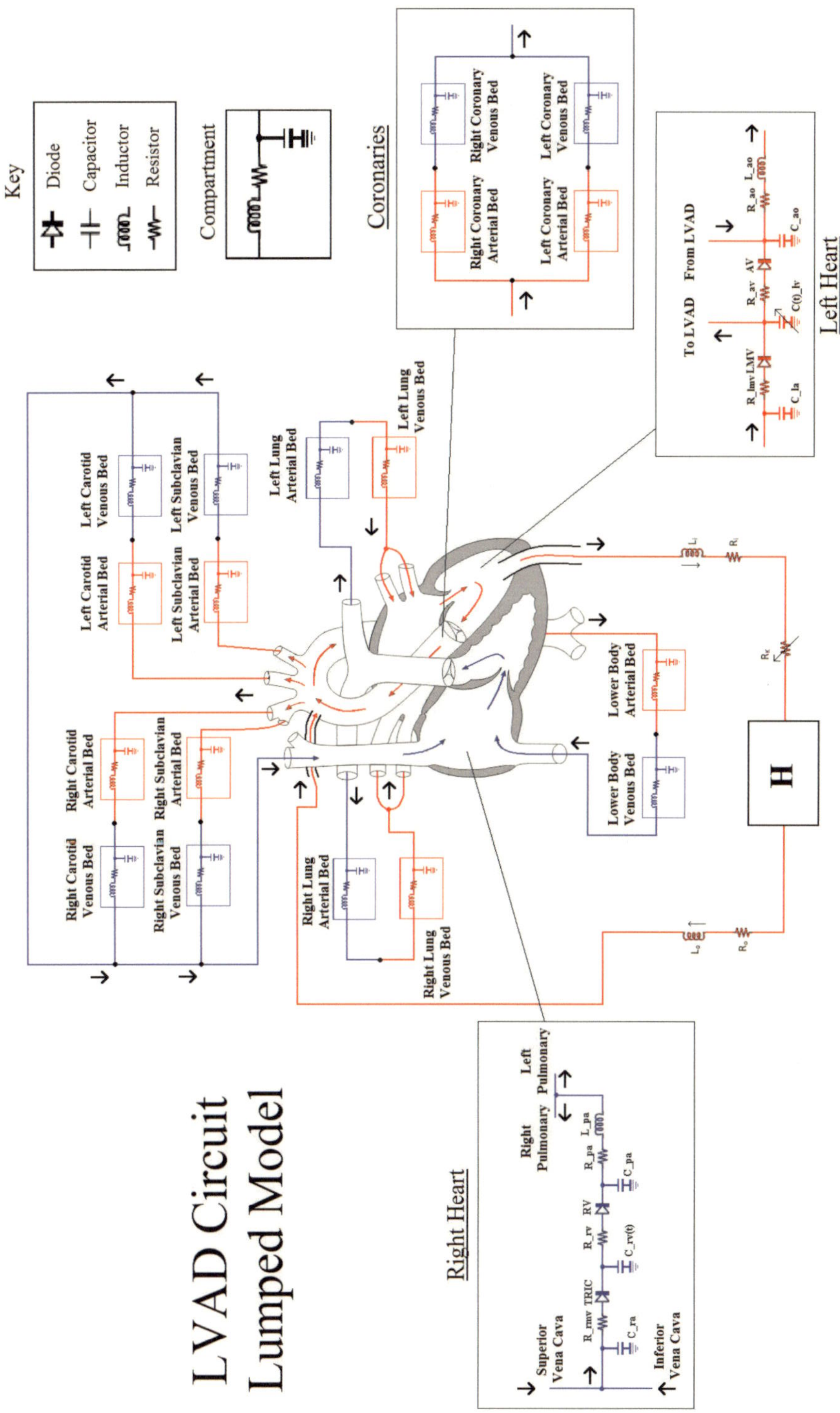

Fig. 7. Multi-DOF electric circuit used to generate the boundary condition waveforms

Figure 8 illustrates the typical geometry of a human aortic arch (Layton et al., 2006) indicating the names of the different branches that stem out of the arch. Figure 9(a)-(c) shows the proposed CFD solid models with the LVAD conduit at (a) normal angle of incidence $\alpha=0°$, (b) intermediate angle of incidence $\alpha=30°$, and shallow angle of incidence $\alpha=60°$. Figure 10(a)-(b) presents the proposed CFD solid models with the LVAD conduit at normal angle of incidence and (a) aortic-to-innominate (IA) bypass and (b) aortic-to-left-carotid (LCA) bypass.

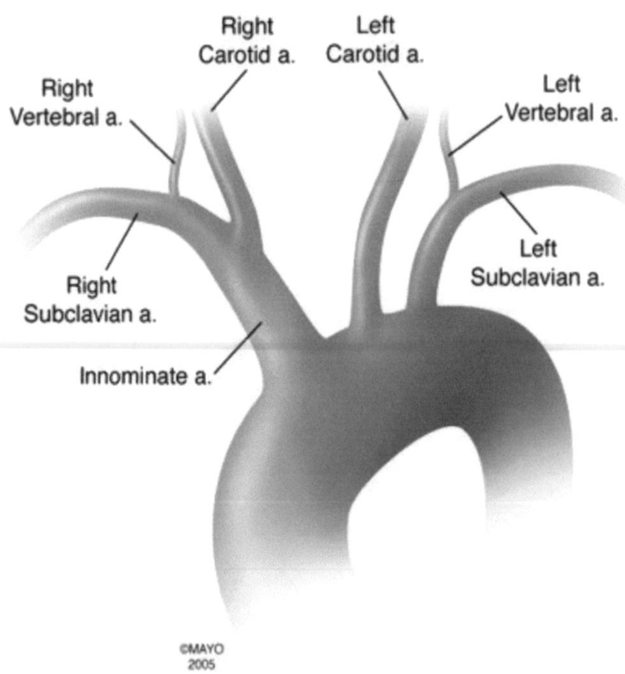

Fig. 8. Most common form of aortic arch in humans (Layton et al., 2006)

Results are presented in the form of velocity vector plots colored by velocity magnitudes around the vicinity of the LVAD cannula anastomosis to the aortic root in Figure 11 (a)-(c) for the different angles of incidence, illustrating the local hemodynamics behavior with pronounced recirculation zones. Table 6 presents the percentage of particle embolization (flow of particles to the left or right Carotid arteries) for the different angles and bypass cases calculated using the particle tracking model by releasing 900 solid, perfectly spherical, particles of diameters 2mm, 4mm and 5 mm, at random locations of the cross-section of the LVAD cannula. These averages reveal significant differences in thrombo-embolization by adjustment of the LVAD inflow cannula and placement of bypass grafts, showing a maximum rate of embolization of close to 50% at shallow angles of incidence in contrast to embolization rates of about 12% at intermediate angles of incidence with bypass implantation. These preliminary results (see Osorio et al., 2009, and El-Zahab et al., 2010) are promising and can potentially offer guidance to surgeons as to the optimal implantation angle and location of the LVAD cannula as well as to the potential implantation of aortic bypass grafts to minimize stroke risk.

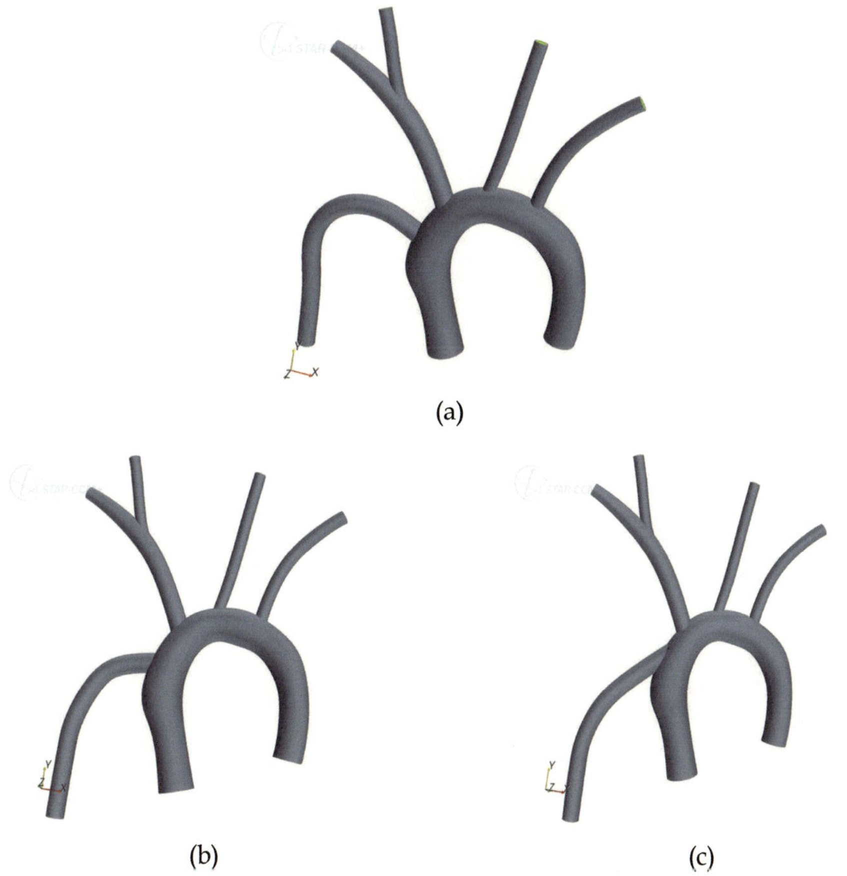

Fig. 9. Solid model of adult aortic arch with LVAD conduit at (a) normal angle of incidence $\alpha=0°$, (b) intermediate angle of incidence $\alpha=30°$, and (c) shallow angle of incidence $\alpha=60°$

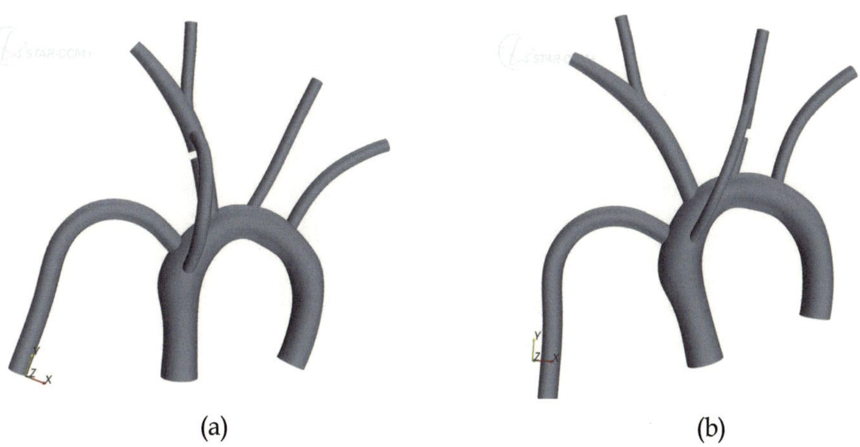

Fig. 10. Solid model of adult aortic arch with LVAD conduit at normal angle of incidence and (a) aortic-to-innominate (IA) bypass and (b) aortic-to-left-carotid (LCA) bypass

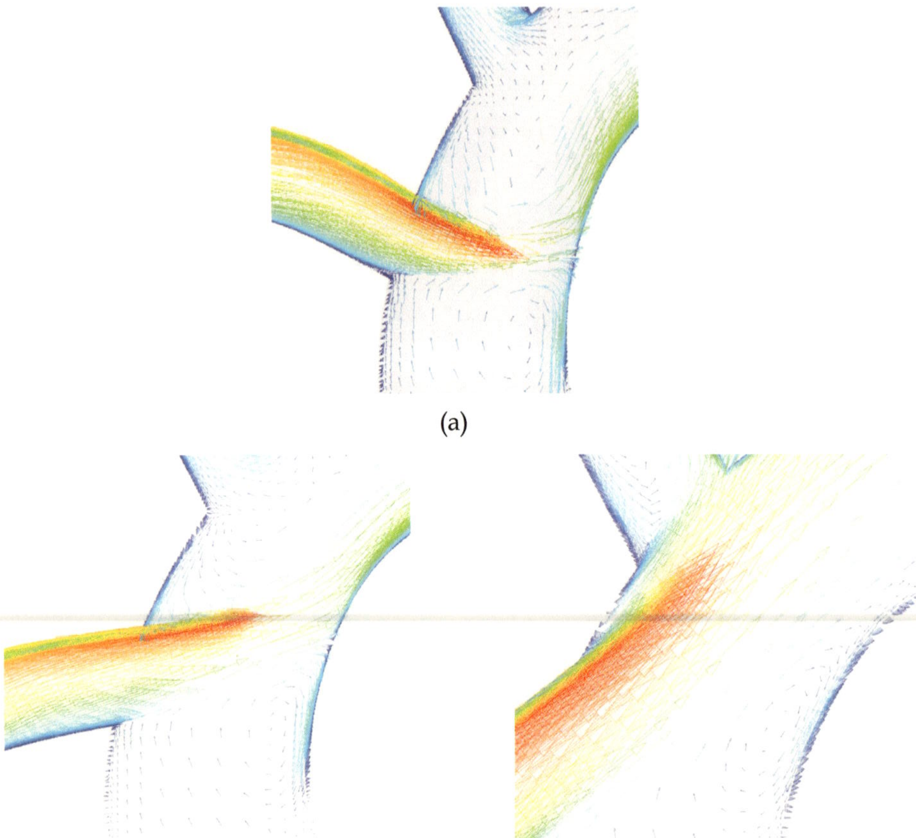

(a)

(b) (c)

Fig. 11. CFD results in the form of vector plots colored by velocity magnitude for LVAD conduit at (a) normal angle of incidence α=0°, (b) intermediate angle of incidence α=30°, and (c) shallow angle of incidence α=60°

Configuration	**Overall [%]**
Standard α=0°	25.60±17.06
IA Bypass α=0°	20.54±10.06
LCA Bypass α=0°	40.93±22.34
Standard α=30°	20.57±9.33
IA Bypass α=30°	14.51±7.62
LCA Bypass α=30°	12.72±5.30
Standard α=60°	47.43±6.44
IA Bypass α=60°	55.66±8.31
LCA Bypass α=60°	34.74±25.98

Table 6. Overall percentage of embolization (thrombi flowing to the LCA and RCA) for the different LVAD conduit angle and bypass configurations

8. Conclusion

In this chapter, we discussed some of the engineering considerations and challenges faced in the design and development of a rotary LVAD. In particular, we presented (1) a current based mathematical model that is appropriate for the design of a feedback controller for the LVAD, (2) an effective algorithm for detection of suction in the left ventricle, and (3) a method for alignment of the outflow cannula of an implanted LVAD to minimize the rate of occurrence of patient trombo-embolic cerebral events.

The model we presented in this chapter is dynamic, 6th order and in state-space format. It represents the combined bio-mechanical system of the LVAD connected to a failing left ventricle with a much reduced elasticity function. The control variable in this model is the pump motor current instead of the pump rotational speed, which so far has been the predominant control variable used in the currently existing models. This model is much more useful for the development of an optimal controller for the LVAD since it avoids solving the inverse problem for determining the pump motor current that yields an already determined optimal pump speed protocol. A method for detecting ventricular suction based on six indices determined from the pump flow signal was also developed. This method is based on the well-known Lagrangian Support Vector Machine technique in pattern recognition. Any feedback controller for the LVAD must take into consideration the detection and avoidance of ventricular suction. Finally, results of a numerical study using Computational Fluid Dynamics and a Lagrangian particle tracking model to predict the path of trombi of different sizes and initial location traveling from the outflow cannula into the circulatory system were presented. This study should be very useful in considering the adjustment of the angle of incidence of the outflow cannula to avoid the occurrence of trombo-embolic cerebral events in LVAD patients.

9. Acknowledgements

This work was supported in part by the US National Science Foundation under grant ECCS-0701365. The authors would like to acknowledge the contributions to the results in sections 2 through 6 of Dr. James F. Antaki (Carnegie Mellon University) and Dr. J. Robert Boston (University of Pittsburgh) and former students Shaohui Chen, Antonio Ferreira and Yih-Chong Yu. The authors would also like to acknowledge the contributions to the results in section 7 of Dr. Alain Kassab (University of Central Florida) and Dr. William DeCampli and Dr. Ricardo Argueta-Morales (Congenital Heart Institute at the Arnold Palmer Hospital for Children in Orlando, Florida).

10. References

Boston, J.; Antaki, J. & Simaan, M. (2003). Hierarchical Control of Hearts Assist Devices. *IEEE Robotics and Automation Magazine*, Vol. 10, No.1, pp. 54-64

Cohen, L. (1995). *Time-Frequency Analysis*. Prentice-Hall, Englewood Cliffs, NJ

Davies, R.; Russo, M.; Hong, K.; O'Byrne, M.; Cork, D.; Moskowitz, A.; Gelijns, A.; Mital, S.; Mosca, R. & Chen, J. (2008). The use of mechanical circulatory support as a bridge to transplantation in pediatric patients: an analysis of the United Network for Organ Sharing database. *The Journal of Thoracic and Cardiovascular Surgery*, Vol. 135, No. 2, pp. 421-427

Dorf, R. & A. Svoboda, J. (2006). *Introduction to Electric Circuits* (7th Edition), John Wiley

Drummond, A.; Onur Dur, O.; Pekkan, K. & Antaki, J. (2008). Simulation of Optimal Surgical Anastomosis of Pediatric Aortic Cannula. *Proceedings of the American Society of Mechanical Engineers Summer Bioengineering Conference (SBC2008),* Paper SBC2008-193064

El-Zahab, Z.; Divo, E. & Kassab, A. (2010). Minimization of the Wall Shear Stress Gradients In Bypass Grafts Anastomoses using Meshless CFD and Genetic Algorithms Optimization. *Computer Methods in Biomechanics and Biomedical Engineering,* Vol. 13, No. 1, pp. 35 – 47

Faragallah, G.; Wang, Y.; Divo, E. & Simaan, M. (2011). A new current-based control model of the combined cardiovascular and rotary left ventricular assist device. *Proceedings of the 2011 American Control Conference,* San Francisco, CA, June 29- July 1, 2011, pp. 4776-4780

Ferreira, A.; Chen, S.; Simaan, M.; Boston, J. & Antaki, J. (2006). A discriminant-analysis-based suction detection system for rotary blood pumps. *Proceedings of 28th IEEE Annual International Conference of Engineering in Medicine and Biology,* New York, NY, 2006, pp. 5382–5385

Frazier, O. & Myers, T.J. (1999) Left Ventricular Assist Systems as a Bridge to Myocardial Recovery. *Annals of Thoracic Surgery,* Vol. 68, pp. 734-741

Gabran, S.; Moussa, W.; Salama, M. & George, C. (2009). Portable real-time support-vector-machine-based automated diagnosis and detection device of narcolepsy episodes. *Proceedings of 31st IEEE Annu. International Conference of Engineering in Medicine and Biology,* Minneapolis, MN, Sep. 2-6, 2009, pp. 903–906

Karantonis, D.; Lovell, N.; Ayre, P.; Mason, D. & Cloherty, S. (2006). Identification and classification of physiologically significant pumping states in an implantable rotary blood pump. *Artificial Organs,* vol. 30, no. 9, pp. 671-679

Karantonis, D.; Cloherty, S.; Lovell, N.; Mason, D.; Salamonsen, R. & Ayre, P. (2008). Noninvasive detection of suction in an implantable rotary blood pump using neural networks. *International Journal of Computation Intelligence and Applications,* vol. 7, pp. 237-247

Layton, K.; Kallmes, D.; Cloft, H.; Lindell, E & Cox, V. (2006). "Bovine Aortic Arch Variant in Humans: Clarification of a Common Misnomer," *American Journal of Neuroradiology.* Vol. 27, pp. 1541-1542

Mason, D.; Hilton, A. & Salamonsen, R. (2008). Reliable Suction Detection for Patients with Rotary Blood Pumps. *The American Society for Artificial Internal Organs (ASAIO) Journal,* Vol. 54, pp. 359-366

Marieb, E. (1994). *Human Anatomy and Physiology.* Pearson Education, San Francisco, CA

Olsen, D. (2000). The History of Continuous-Flow Blood Pumps. *Artificial Organs,* Vol. 24, No. 6, pp. 401-404

Oshikawa, M.; Araki, K.; Endo, G.; Anai, H. & Sato, M. (2000). Sensorless controlling method for a continuous flow left ventricular assist device. *Artificial Organs,* vol. 24, no. 8, pp. 600-605

Osorio, A.; Kassab, A.; Divo, E.; Argueta-Morales, R. & DeCampli, W. (2009). Computational Fluid Dynamics Analysis of Surgical Adjustement of Ventricular Assist Device Implantation to Minimize Stroke Risk, *American Society of Mechanical Engineers,* paper IMECE2009-12813

Poirier, V. (1997). The LVAD: A Case Study. *The Bridge,* Vol. 27, pp. 14-20

Russo, M.; Hong, K.; Davies, R.; Chen, J.; Sorabella, R.; Ascheim, D.; Williams, M.; Gelijns, A.; Stewart, A.; Argenziano, M. & Naka, Y. (2009). Posttransplant survival is not diminished in heart transplant recipients bridged with implantable left ventricular assist devices. *The Journal of Thoracic and Cardiovascular Surgery,* Vol. 138, No. 6, pp.1425-1432

Schmid, C.; Weyand, M.; Nabavi, D.; Hammel, D.; Deng, M.; Ringelstein, E. & Scheld, H. (1998). Cerebral and systemic embolization during left ventricular support with the Novacor N100 device. *The Annals of Thoracic Surgery,* Vol. 65, No. 6, pp.1703-1710

Shahcheraghi, N.; Dwyer, H.; Cheer, A.Y.; Barakat, A.I. & Rutaganira, T. (2002). Unsteady and Three-Dimensional Simulation of Blood Flow in the Human Aortic Arch. *American Society of Mechanical Engineers Journal of Biomechanical Engineering,* Vol. 124, No. 4, pp. 378-387.

Tokuda, Y.; Song, M-H; Ueda, Y.; Usui, A.; Akita, T.; Yoneyama, S. & Maruyama, S. (2008). Three-dimensional numerical simulation of blood flow in the aortic arch during cardiopulmonary bypass. *European Journal of Cardio-thoracic Surgery,* Vol.33, pp. 164-167

Schima, H.; Trubel, W.; Moritz, A.; Wieselthaler, G.; Stohr, H.; Thoma, H.; Losert, U. & Wolner, E. (1992). Noninvasive Monitoring of Rotary Blood Pumps: Necessity, Possibilities, and Limitations. *Artificial Organs,* Vol. 14, No. 2, pp. 195-202

Simaan, M. A.; Ferreira, A.; Chen, S.; Antaki, J. & Galati, D. (2009). A Dynamical State-Space Representation and Performance Analysis of A Feedback-Controlled Rotary Left Ventricular Assist Device. *IEEE Transactions on Control Systems Technology,* Vol.17, No. 1, (January 2009), pp. 15-28

Simaan, M. A. (2009). *Rotary Heart Assist Devices.* Chapter 79 in Springer Handbook of Automation, Nof (ED). pp. 1409-1422

Sitaram, R.; Lee, S.; Ruiz, S.; Rana, M.; Veit, R. & Birbaumer, N. (2011) Real-time support vector classification and feedback of multiple emotional brain states. *Journal of NeuroImage,* Vol. 56, pp. 753-765

Stergiopulos, N.; Meister, J. & Westerhof, N. (1996a). Determinants of Stroke Volume and Systolic and Diastolic Aortic Pressure. *American Journal of Physiology,* Vol. 270, No. 6, 1996, pp. H2050-H2059

Stergiopulos, N.; Westerhof, B.; Meister, J. & Westerhof, N. (1996b). The Four Element Windkessel Model. *Proceedings of the 18th IEEE Engineering in Medicine and Biology Annual International Conference,* Amsterdam, Holland, 1996, pp. 1715-1716

Suga, H. & Sagawa, K. (1974). Instantaneous Pressure-Volume Relationships and Their Ratio in the Excised, Supported Canine Left Ventricle. *Circulation Research,* Vol. 35, No. 1, 1974, pp. 117-126

Thoennissen, N.; Allroggen, A.; Ritter, M.; Dittrich, R.; Schmid, C.; Schmid, H.; Ringelstein, E. & Nabavi, D.G. (2006). Influence of Inflammation and Pump Dynamic on Cerebral Microembolization in Patients with Continuous-Flow DeBakey LVAD. *American Society of Internal Artificial Organs (ASAIO)* , Vol. 52, No. 3, pp.243-247

Vollkron, M.; Schima, H.; Huber, L.; Benkowski, R.; Morello, G. & Wieselthaler, G. (2004). Development of a Suction Detection System for Axial Blood Pumps. *Artificial Organs,* Vol. 28, No. 8, 2004, pp. 709-716

Vollkron, M.; Schima, H.; Huber, L.; Benkowski, R.; Morello, G. & Wieselthaler, G. (2006). Advanced Suction Detection for an Axial Flow Pump. *Artificial Organs*, Vol. 30, No. 9, 2006, pp. 665-670

Wang, Y.; Faragallah, G.; Divo, E. & Simaan, M. (2011). Detection of Ventricular Suction in an Implantable Rotary Blood Pump Using Support Vector Machines. *Proceedings of the 33rd IEEE Annual International Conference of Engineering in Medicine and Biology*, Boston, MA, 2011

Yu, Y-C.; Boston, J.; Simaan, M. & Antaki, J. (1998). Estimation of Systemic Vascular Bed Parameters for Artificial Heart Control. *IEEE Transactions on Automatic Control*, Vol. 43, No. 6, 1998, pp. 765-778

Yuhki, A.; Hatoh, E.; Nogawa, M.; Miura, M.; Shimazaki, Y. & Takatani, S. (1999). Detection of Suction and Regurgitation of the Implantable Centrifugal Pump Based on the Motor Current Waveform Analysis and its Application to Optimization of the Pump Flow. *Artificial Organs*, 1999, Vol. 23, pp. 532-537

3

Evaluation of Cardiac Function after VAD Implantation

John Terrovitis, Eleni Tseliou, Stavros Drakos and John Nanas
3rd Department of Cardiology, University of Athens
Greece

1. Introduction

Heart failure constitutes a major health problem with a current prevalence of over 5.8 million in the USA and over 23 million worldwide. (Lloyd-Jones, 2010) During the last decades a dramatic increase in the number of heart failure patients and hospitalizations was observed (Curtis et al., 2008) with an incidence of more than 550,000 annually in the USA and a lifetime risk of 20%. Although prevalence increases with age, heart failure can also affect young patients (Lloyd-Jones, 2010; Levy et al, 2002; Lloyd-Jones et al, 2002). It is also estimated that 10% from all HF patients have reached advanced stages of the disease, which is characterized by development of symptoms refractory to standard treatment, often requiring prolonged hospitalizations, intravenous vasoactive medication and diuretics and ultimately, consideration of mechanical support (Ammar et al., 2007).

Despite the therapeutic advances in the recent decades and the improvement in prognosis (drugs that counteract neurohormonal activation, devices that prevent or treat lethal arrhythmias and correct dyssynchrony), advanced heart failure remains a lethal clinical syndrome. Mortality rate for patients who had to be hospitalized due to heart failure deterioration is approaching 75% at 5 years; for end stage patients it is almost 80% (Ammar et al., 2007).

Cardiac transplantation is currently the best available treatment of advanced heart failure, but it is available to fewer than 2500 patients in the United States each year, when approximately 5–10 people are on the waiting list for each transplant taking place (Taylor et al., 2009). In addition, hundreds of thousands of patients who have severe end-stage heart failure are not eligible for a heart transplant due to concomitant multisystem disease, uncontrolled diabetes, continued tobacco use, or psychosocial limitations; however their condition continuously deteriorates.

The limitations of medical therapy in advanced stage heart failure, the lack of donor organ availability, and the large number of patients who do not qualify for transplantation due to contraindications, have spurred interest in mechanical circulatory support (MCS). Since the mid 1980s, for patients experiencing recurrent hospitalizations for heart failure decompensation despite optimal treatment and manifesting symptoms or signs of progressive end organ dysfunction, mechanical support of the circulation with Ventricular Assist Devices (VADs) has a well established and continuously expanding role (Stevenson & Rose, 2003). In addition to short term support of critically ill patients with appropriate devices, long term Left Ventricular Assist Devices (LVADs) have been approved for transplant candidates as bridge to transplantation or for patients suitable for destination therapy as permanent treatment (Miller et al., 2007; Slaughter et al., 2009). There is now compelling evidence that prolonged unloading of the left ventricle with the use of an LVAD is associated with structural reverse remodeling (Mancini et al., 1998; Drakos et al., 2007) that can be accompanied by significant functional improvement (Dandel et al., 2005). Therefore, a new, although relatively rare indication for mechanical support is emerging, namely bridge to recovery (Hon & Yacoub, 2003).

However, before the use of ventricular assist devices as a "bridge to myocardial improvement" or complete recovery becomes feasible, reliable methods to detect complete recovery need to be developed. The optimal time for device removal in these cases need also to be determined, in order to guarantee safe and effective weaning from the device and long-term clinical stability without mechanical support. These tasks are by no means trivial, since the operation of the assist device makes evaluation of most of the currently available indices (echocardiographic parameters, biomarkers) difficult.

In addition, the continuously expanding role of LVADs as destination therapy mandates the evaluation of device and cardiac function at regular intervals, in order to detect system malfunction, thrombosis, or complications such as progression of valvular or right heart disease. Changes in patient symptoms or hemodynamics should prompt a thorough investigation of the function of both the pump and the supported heart. Knowledge of the underlying functional reserve of the patient's heart is necessary, in order to estimate the urgency of a device exchange procedure, in case of mechanical failure.

For these reasons, evaluation of cardiac function during mechanical support has emerged as one of the key factors for the optimal management of this group of patients. Many different approaches, involving both established clinical modalities such as echocardiography together with advanced techniques at the cellular and molecular level are being applied.

2. Remodeling: Potentially reversible alterations

It is important to recognize that HF is a syndrome rather than a primary diagnosis with many potential etiologies, diverse clinical features, and numerous clinical subsets. It is a progressive disorder with principal manifestation a change in the geometry and structure of the LV; the chamber dilates and/or hypertrophies and becomes more spherical—a process referred to as cardiac remodeling. Apart from the anatomic changes, the biology of the cardiac myocyte, and the structure and volume of myocyte and nonmyocyte components of the myocardium, are also affected.

There are two major categories of unfavorable alterations that occur in failing myocardium; these that occur in the volume and structure of cardiac myocytes and these that occur in the volume and composition of the extracellular matrix. As far as the first is concerned, increasing evidence suggests that progressive myocyte loss, through both necrotic and apoptotic cell death due to excessive adrenergic stimulation, (Josue et al., 1907) takes place in the myocardium of patients with advanced heart failure (Mann et al., 1992). The loss of functional myocardial tissue increases the work of the normal myocardial cells, leading to hypertrophy in an attempt to cope with the higher load, by increasing the number of sarcomeres. However, the chronically increased rate of energy consumption puts the cells of the hypertrophied and failing heart in an energy-starved state (Katz, 1988). Endomyocardial biopsies taken from the hearts of patients with congestive heart failure have shown a correlation between decreased ATP content and impaired contraction and relaxation. (Bashore et al., 1987). Abnormalities in calcium homeostasis were also found in failing cardiomyocytes leading to abnormal contractile function and force-frequency relationships.

In addition, there are several important changes that occur within the extracellular matrix of the myocardium (Thomas et al., 1998; Tyagi et al., 1996; Tyagi et al., 1996; Li et al., 1998), with fibrosis being the most widely recognized. Fibrosis due to excessive deposition of fibrillar collagen occurs around intramyocardial blood vessels and as replacement of lost myocytes. A family of collagenolytic enzymes, matrix metalloproteinases (MMPs), becomes also activated within the failing myocardium (Thomas et al., 1998; Tyagi et al., 1996; Li et al., 1998). Activation of MMPs leads to progressive degradation of the extracellular matrix, which in turn leads to realignment (slippage) of myocyte bundles and/or individual myocytes within the LV wall, and thus accounts for the LV wall thinning and the dilation that occurs in heart failure.

These alterations in the biochemical composition of the myocardium impose several de novo mechanical burdens on the failing heart. Perhaps the most obvious problem that occurs in the remodeled ventricle is the increase in LV end-diastolic volume, and hence end-diastolic wall stress. As the load on the ventricle at end-diastole contributes importantly to the afterload of the ventricle at the onset of systole, LV dilation by itself will increase the work of the ventricle, and hence the oxygen demand. The increase in wall thinning along with the increase in afterload created by LV dilation leads to a functional afterload mismatch that may further contribute to a decrease in forward cardiac output and shifts the end-diastolic pressure-volume relation (EDPVR) towards larger volumes (Burkhoff et al.; 1988) Moreover, the high end-diastolic wall stress may even lead to episodic hypoperfusion of the subendocardium with resultant worsening of LV function (Vatner et al., 1988, Shannon et al., 1993; LeGrice et al., 1995; Givertz et al., 1998).

Accordingly, there has been significant interest in developing therapeutic interventions to prevent and reverse these processes of adverse remodeling. Both angiotensin-converting enzyme inhibitors and nitroglycerin have been shown to attenuate ventricular enlargement after myocardial infarction, suggesting, at least in part, that reduction of wall stress may be an important factor for amelioration of remodeling (Jugdutt et al., 1988; Pfeffer et al., 1988). In addition, chronic ß-blocker therapy reduces ventricular mass and normalizes left ventricular shape in patients with heart failure (Hall S et al., 1994). Thus, evidence from pharmacological interventions that target neurohormonal activation and hemodynamic stress in heart failure suggested that the remodeling process may be reversed to some degree, although to a limited extent; this knowledge challenged the notion that ventricular dilation due to remodeling in advanced heart failure is an irreversible process. More importantly, this generated the hypothesis that ventricular assist devices, which have been used in critically ill patients awaiting heart transplantation, may reverse the remodeling changes to a greater extent, even up to the level of complete recovery, since they can provide profound hemodynamic unloading of the left ventricle, unparallel to the respective achieved by combination of drug treatment.

3. Principles of LVAD operation

The Artificial Heart Program of the National Heart, Lung, and Blood Institute, chartered in 1964, sponsored and initialized the development of mechanical cardiac-support devices (Hogness et al., 1991). The first goal was to develop a device for the temporary support of a patient with terminal heart failure until a donor organ could be found. This strategy has become a daily reality in transplantation centers worldwide since the approval by the Food and Drug Administration (FDA) of the pneumatically driven left ventricular assist devices as a bridge to transplantation in 1994 and of the self-contained, vented electric devices for the same purpose in 1998 (Mancini et al., 1998; McCarthy et al., 1998; DeRose et al., 1997).

Candidates for left ventricular or biventricular assist devices were patients eligible for transplantation with signs of near circulatory collapse, generalized debilitation, or end-organ deterioration, in order to improve their eligibility for transplantation and their chances for survival. The last decade, pulsatile left ventricular assist devices (LVADs) have been replaced by devices which continuously expel blood volume from within the failing left ventricle into the aorta. In 2008, the Food and Drug Administration approved the use of the continuous flow LVAD (HeartMate II) in patients who were candidates for bridge to transplantation and in 2010 for destination therapy (Thoratec, 2009).

4. Types of LVADs

The first LVADs were pulsatile volume displacement pumps. The main ones are the Heartmate I, the Thoratec paracorporeal VAD (PVAD, that can be used to support both ventricles), the Berlin Heart (paracorporeal, suitable for biventricular support), Novacor and the Cardiowest total artificial heart.

The Heartmate I has been widely used and inserted in over 5000 patients. It's flow pattern is pulsatile, similar to the normal circulation and can pump 4–10 l/min. Valves in the inflow and outflow cannulas ensure unidirectional flow through the system. A unique inner surface texture negates the use of anticoagulation and only antiplatelet therapy is needed. This device was used in the landmark REMATCH trial and was the first one to be approved as destination therapy.

Although pulsatile pumps provide excellent hemodynamic support, they have limitations, particularly their large size (hence needing extensive surgical dissection and patients with adequate body size), noisy operation, and importantly, limited long-term durability (Lahpor, 2009).

Continuous flow or second-generation axial flow pumps are being increasingly used during the last decade, as LVADs. These are continuous-flow rotary pumps that have only one moving part, the rotor, unlike the first-generation devices, and hence are expected to be more durable. The more frequently used ones are the Heartmate II, Berlin Heart Incor, the Jarvik 2000 and the MicroMed-DeBakey VAD.

The HeartMate II pump (Thoratec Corp.) is the only continuous-flow pump currently approved as a bridge to transplantation and destination therapy. This device can be operated at a pump speed between 8,000 to 12,000 revolutions/min (RPM), generating flow rates up to 10 l/min. In comparison to the first-generation Heartmate I device, it is one-seventh its size and one-quarter its weight. Over 3000 patients have had a Heartmate II implanted and is the most widely used second-generation device.

The mean duration of support reported for these continuous flow, rotary pumps is longer compared with the first-generation devices (166–236 vs. 50–60 days) (El-Banayosy et al., 2000). The incidence of thrombo-embolic events in HeartMate II patients is in most studies comparable with the Heart- Mate I with annual ischemic stroke rates ranging from 3 to 6% and for transient ischemic attacks from 1 to 4% (Strüber et al., 2008). Hemorrhagic stroke rates tend to be higher (2–3%), probably due to the need for anticoagulation. A somewhat higher neurologic complication rate has been reported with the use of another nonpulsatile device, the Micromed DeBakey VAD (stroke rate 15–18%).

Newer implantable (nonpulsatile with magnetic bearings) pumps, such as the VentrAssist, DuraHeart and HeartWare, currently under evaluation in clinical trials, may combine the advantages of even smaller size with longer durabilty.

5. Alteration of cardiac hemodynamics by LVAD support

The primary action of an LVAD is to provide volume and pressure unloading of the LV, while simultaneously restoring systemic blood pressure and blood flow to the peripheral organs. At the same time, LVAD support eliminates the need for administration of potentially toxic pressors and inotropes (McCarthy et al., 1995; Frazier et al., 1996). With most LVADs , this is achieved by withdrawing blood from the left ventricle (most often) or left atrium and returning it to the arterial system, providing in this way profound LV pressure and volume unloading. This also results in reductions in pulmonary venous and arterial pressures and pulmonary vascular resistance (Klotz et al., 2004). The normalization of blood pressure and cardiac output, improves perfusion to all body organs, which results in improved autonomic function and normalization of the neurohormonal and cytokine milieu that is present in heart failure (McCarthy et al., 1995).

Heart failure is considered a systemic disease that affects many organs because of hypoperfusion and the abnormal neurohormonal and cytokine stimulation; normalization of the latter by LVADs promotes recovery not only of the heart but of all peripheral organs as well (Levine & Levine , 1990). Not all effects of LVAD support, however, are beneficial. LVADs provide pressure and volume unloading only to the LV. In the face of increased cardiac output, the right ventricle (RV) (often diseased due to a cardiomyopathy process or due to chronic pressure and volume overload) can become volume overloaded and unable to accommodate the resultant flow (Ochiai et al., 2002). In addition, excessive unloading of the LV provokes RV dysfunction, by shifting the interventricular septum to the left. This increases RV diameter, right ventricular wall stress and consequently RV afterload. As a result, RV distention and failure occur in as many as 20% to 30% of LVAD recipients (Ochiai et al., 2002). More specifically, RV and LV are connected in series and interact with each other hemodynamically, due to the anatomic coupling provided by the shared interventricular septum and common muscle fibers. The impact of LV support by an LVAD on RV geometry, hemodynamics and function can be complex. The reduction of LV filling pressures by the LVAD can decrease substantially RV afterload and in that way improve RV function. On the same time, the LVAD can increase venous return to the RV (by increasing cardiac output), therefore RV operates with a higher preload. An LVAD that excessively unloads the LV can produce a leftward septal shift. This can potentially improve RV filling, however at the same time it reduces substantially the systolic LV contribution to RV contraction, through dyscoordination of interventricular septal motion, and the overall effect may be a significant deterioration of RV function. RV failure occurring after LVAD implantation can be treated with inotropic agents and pulmonary vasodilators, while at the same time optimization of the LVAD function (adjustment of RPM in case of continuous flow devices) is mandatory. Despite these measures, simultaneous right ventricular support is required in many cases.

During the previous decade, pulsatile LVADs were dominating clinical use; however, in the recent years nonpulsatile devices are by far more frequently used in the clinical practice, and next-generation devices in development are also based on the same principal of continuous flow (axial or centrifugal). Although these novel devices are, as already mentioned, smaller, more durable and reliable, more energy efficient, less thrombogenic, and less surgically traumatic to implant, they do not generate normal pulsatile flow. Although there is considerable data that long term non-pulsatile flow does not have detrimental effects on end-organ function, little is known about the consequences of lack of pulsatility on reverse remodeling. Klotz et al investigated the hemodynamic effects during long-term support with nonpulsatile and pulsatile LVADs; they found that LV pressure unloading was similar between these 2 types of LVADs, whereas LV volume unloading was significantly more pronounced with a pulsatile device (Klotz et al., 2004). The significance of this difference is not known.

Thohan et al showed that although there are differences between these two classes of devices with regard to magnitude of unloading, both forms of support were equally effective in normalizing cell size and tumor necrosis factor-alfa levels (Thohan et al., 2005).

Most recently, Bartoli et al studied the effect of continuous vs pulsatile devices on cardiac hemodynamics, in a bovine model of left ventricular heart failure. Their data revealed that continuous unloading diminished energy requirements during cardiac cycle to non-physiological levels, particularly at higher levels of support. During increasing levels of continuous unloading, the variation between end-systolic and end-diastolic pressures diminished significantly, volumes and pressures decreased to non-physiologically low values and resulted in chronic closure of the aortic valve. On the other hand, pulsatile flow during left ventricular support, despite similar reduction in left ventricular end diastolic volumes, preserved a normal range of physiologic pressures. Therefore, continuous unloading dramatically reduces cardiac metabolic demands to values that are not normally observed in mammals; the significance of this observation for cardiac function during long term support is still unknown (Bartoli et al., 2010).

However, there are also physiological limitations to the function of pulsatile VADs. Klotz et al. demonstrated that with pulsatile LVADs device ejection is not generally coordinated with ventricular contraction and this device–heart dyssynchrony may paradoxically increase afterload. This is a result of the fact that native left ventricular contraction can occur at a phase when both the inlet valve of the device and the native aortic valve are closed (the latter due to higher aortic than ventricular pressure). This results in isometric ventricular contraction, which is energy demanding and non-efficient and can cause excessive stretching of the myocardium, particularly in the presence of systemic hypertension, which can occur following left ventricular assist device insertion, particularly of the pulsatile type. Regurgitation of the inlet valve of the left ventricular assist device can also result in systolic and diastolic stretching of the myocardium. On the other hand continuous-type flow pumps, are not subject to such dyssynchrony. While the degree of pressure unloading is similar to pulsatile LVADs, systemic arterial pressure is not increased to the same extent with continuous flow LVADs. In addition, although flow across the aortic valve is evident in less than 40% of the patients with continuous flow LVADs, as already mentioned, the absence of inflow and outflow device valves allows forward flow during each left ventricular ejection, even if this occurs with low systolic pressures. In that way, the afterload of the native ventricle is kept low continuously.

These fundamental, functional differences between the pulsatile and nonpulsatile LVADs are crucial especially for the evaluation of cardiac function after device implantation, as it will be later shown.

6. Reverse remodeling

One of the earliest recognized changes of patients' hearts supported by an LVAD until transplantation was the reduction of the size of the cardiac silhouette on chest radiographs, observed immediately before transplantation possibly due to the unloading of the dilated heart. In addition, retrospective analysis of echocardiograms showed that after a short term period of LVAD support, LV end diastolic diameter decreased significantly (6.81 to 5.39mm), with corresponding increases in ejection fraction (11% to 22%). Echocardiographic studies performed in the pre-implant period and at explantation at the time of transplantation in 20 patients, in order to further investigate the effect of unloading on left ventricular function, showed a significant decrease in LV end-diastolic volume, LV end-systolic volume, left atrial volume, and an increase in LV ejection fraction (Thohan et al., 2005).

LV pressure-volume relationships were also evaluated in LVAD supported hearts after explantation and a shift towards normal was observed, suggesting that multiple favorable alterations at the cellular, tissue and whole organ level had occurred, described with the general term reverse remodeling (Levin et al., 1995). Although the hearts did not return to completely normal size, an average time of 30.8 days was needed in order for the reverse remodeling to be observed, while at 90 days most of the process was completed in this patient cohort (Madigan et al., 2001). In contrast, reverse remodeling of RV in LVAD supported hearts was not observed, suggesting that reverse structural remodeling is primarily mediated by the profound hemodynamic unloading and not only by normalized neurohormonal milieu, as previously already mentioned (Barbone et al., 2001). Another explanation of this discrepancy in favorable outcome between the LV and the RV might be the RV dysfunction induced by excessive LV unloading, as previously explained. It is of interest that when an RVAD is implanted in the RV, changes in the RV End Diastolic Pressure - Volume relationships are comparable with those observed in the LV of LVAD supported hearts (Klotz et al., 2005).

In addition to the effects on structure, the LVAD supported hearts on average exhibited reduced left ventricular trabeculae length, diameter, and mass as compared to the medically managed hearts. LVAD support, led also to increased contractile strength, faster time to peak concentration and reduced time to 50% relaxation in isolated cardiomyocytes (Dipla et al., 1998). Myocytes also exhibited improved contractile responses to increased frequency of stimulation, an effect blunted in end-stage heart failure. This was paralleled by normalization of b-adrenergic receptor density and reversal of RyR2 hyperphosphorylation (Marx et al., 2000). In addition, Klotz S et al. showed that LVAD support was associated with a significant increase in total and especially cross linked collagen deposition in LV myocardium (Klotz et al., 2005). The levels and activity of matrix metalloproteinases tended to decrease following LVAD support. Again, a similar structural reverse remodeling was not generally observed in the RV (Barbone et al., 2001).

7. Bridge to recovery

Even in the first Bridge to Transplantation trials, a small but increasing number of cases was noted where after a certain time of support the ventricular function improved sufficiently to allow consideration of removal of the device. Some patients, after explantation, were discharged without requiring heart transplantation and the idea of bridge to recovery emerged (Levin et al., 1994). In 1996, Levin et al. described for the first time the explantation of an LVAD in a 19-year-old man who had advanced heart failure caused by idiopathic dilated cardiomyopathy. Following LVAD support for 183 days the device was explanted but unfortunately, the heart redilated soon after the explantation procedure; ejection fraction worsened, and the patient died of heart failure (Levin et al., 1996).

In 1998 Mancini et al published a retrospective review of a total of 111 LVAD patients, evaluated for cardiac recovery. Only 5 successful explantations were identified (Mancini et al., 1998).

Low rate of recovery (9%) was published from Maybaum et al. in a study that included 67 patients supported by LVAD. Simon et al reported recovery in 11% of the non ischemic patients and only 2.5% in the ischemic population in a study of 154 LVAD patients (Simon et al., 2005).

However, in other series results have been more promising. In patients with acute myocarditis, it is well known that the combination of profound mechanical cardiac unloading and the appropriate therapy allows complete recovery and weaning from LVAD support in many cases (Farrar et al., 2002; Grinda et al., 2004). Muller et al reported a higher percentage of recovery and explantation in 17 patients with dilated cardiomyopathy; In 5 out of the 17 (29%) patients after 160 days of mechanical support the LVADs were successfully explanted and patients maintained normal cardiac function for 51 to 592 days (Muller et al., 1997)

The most promising results were reported by Yacoub and co-workers, with the use of a protocol combining mechanical unloading of the left ventricle with an optimum medical treatment at maximal tolerated doses, including β2-receptor stimulation. With this approach, in a carefully selected patient population of dilated cardiomyopathy patients, 11 of 15 (73%) demonstrated cardiac recovery sufficient to undergo successful device explantation, with 100% and 89% cumulative rates of freedom from recurrent HF at 1 and 4 years, respectively (Birks EJ et al., 2006). This study was conducted using the first-generation, pulsatile HeartMate XVE device. Interestingly, the same group demonstrated better results for quality of life in the bridge to recovery group 3.6 years after the LVAD removal, compared to the bridge to transplantation patients and even to transplanted patients (George et al., 2008).

Recently, the same investigators presented data supporting the feasibility of sustainable myocardial recovery using a continuous flow LVAD. They published the results of 19 non ischemic cardiac failure patients, who underwent implantation of a HeartMate II pump as a bridge to recovery. The successful explantation rate was 63.2% at 2 years. Estimated survival without heart failure recurrence was 83.3% at 1 and 3 years (Birks et al., 2011).

Nevertheless, results from other, larger series of DCM patients were not similarly encouraging, either as far as explantation rates or sustainability of recovery is concerned. All these studies should be interpreted with caution, since patient selection, devices and pharmacological protocols varied considerably. However, if bridge to recovery ever becomes an acceptable indication for LVAD therapy, the need for validated protocols for left ventricular function assessment during support will become even more pressing.

8. Destination therapy

After the landmark REMATCH trial, LVAD use as destination therapy became an accepted indication, for patients with advanced stage heart failure and contraindications to cardiac transplantation. Recently, even better results have been achieved with the new generation continuous flow pumps. Although destination therapy is considered permanent, there are many reasons why assessment of cardiac function should be performed regularly. Right ventricular failure can manifest even many years after LVAD implantation. Aortic valve disease can also progress after many years of support and can have important hemodynamic consequences.

9. Evaluation protocols

Despite these promising results, the clinical reality shows that the actual percentage of true complete myocardial recovery leading to successful weaning and device explantation is low. Therefore, identification of these patients is a challenging but absolutely necessary task, in order to avoid inappropriate device explantations and risking significant patient morbidity and mortality.

Several groups have used protocols to assess functional performance of the native heart, under reduced levels of support.

Mancini et al. attempted to define criteria in order to identify potential candidates for LVAD explantation. They analyzed a retrospective cohort of 111 LVAD supported patients. They were able to find 5 patients that successfully underwent explantation of the LVAD. However, in 4 heart failure recurred, 2 died and 2 underwent new LVAD implantation (interestingly, in one of them recovery was again observed). Only one patient remained clinically stable with good LV function at 15 months after explantation. Subsequently, they applied strict criteria in a prospective cohort of 39 patients, supported by the pulsatile HeartMAte XVE system. They used cardiopulmonary exercise testing, right heart catheterization, echocardiographic, and data from the LVAD sensor. Measurements were obtained during stress in the automated mode of the device (full support), during down titration of the level of support, and during exercise at a fixed low rate (20bpm). Adequate peak VO2 (>20ml/kg/min) and cardiac output (10 l/min), the presence of an open aortic valve during each cardiac cycle and maintenance of normal-size left ventricle with normal fractional shortening after completion of the exercise protocol at low support levels were criteria for LVAD explantation. Significant clinical recovery occurred in only one of the prospectively studied patients. Limitations of this protocol were the relatively short period of support and the rapid weaning protocol used, that may have not allowed adaptation of patient's hemodynamics and neurohormonal status to the higher demands of the low-support status (Mancini et al., 1998b).

Other studies have confirmed the results of low rates of ventricular recovery, as well as the recurrence of heart failure frequently with the need of LVAD re-implantation, a process often referred to as recurrent remodeling (El-Banayosy et al., 2001; Helman et al., 2000). A common finding in these studies was the higher rate of recovery in patients with idiopathic dilated cardiomyopathy.

Muller et al used a more progressive and prolonged weaning procedure in order to identify truly recovered patients. They evaluated 17 patients with IDC under support with pulsatile pumps (Novacor or HeartMate XVE). They used echocardiography after 4 minutes of complete withdrawal of support to assess complete myocardial recovery (stable EF and ventricular dimensions at normal or nearly normal levels). Subsequently, they put patients with signs of substantial recovery on fixed, asynchronous mode of support for 3 consecutive weeks, in order to test the stability of cardiac function. The fixed-rate mode leads to a dissociation in the coordination between cardiac ejection and optimum filling of the pump, a discrepancy that tends to increase left ventricular afterload. When this occurs, synchronization between heart and pump is random at best. Investigators were able to identify 5 patients who underwent successful LVAD explantation. All remained clinically stable for a period of 51 to 592 days. The approach of keeping patients at increased demands (high afterload) before removal is intriguing, because it could potentially identify those at risk for rapid deterioration. Unfortunately no data about hemodynamics, echocardiography parameters or exercise tolerance at the completion of this testing period were provided. Nevertheless, 29% of the IDC patients were successfully weaned. Importantly, all patients in this study were under maximum pharmacological treatment. Another interesting observation was that, according to the findings of this study, longer periods of support (ventricular unloading for more than 100 days) may have actually been detrimental to recovery and may have contributed to myocyte atrophy (Muller et al., 1997).

Maybaum et al. in a prospective, multicenter, observational study used a slightly different clinical protocol for the evaluation of recovery in 67 patients supported by pulsatile pumps. Monthly assessments were performed including resting echocardiogram at full and reduced (output of 4 l/min) LVAD support, and cardiopulmonary exercise testing in ambulatory patients. Patients with LV ejection fraction (LVEF) 40% at reduced device support underwent dobutamine echocardiography with simultaneous hemodynamic monitoring. Complete recovery leading to LVAD explantation was observed only in the 9% (6/67) of the patients enrolled. Some interesting observations were made in this study. All patients that were successfully weaned demonstrated high contractile reserve on the dobutamine echocardiogram (mean EF of 60±10% at peak dobutamine dose), suggesting that contractile reserve may be a valid clinical tool for studying LV function under LVAD support. At the lowest rate of support, recovered patients had a wedge pressure of 8.5±4.5 versus 15±5.7 mm Hg of those that did not demonstrate similar improvement, indicating that a normal wedge pressure under partial support can be an important indicator of genuine recovery. Four out of 6 of the recovered patients had a short history of heart failure (2 acute myocarditis, 1 recent myocardial infarction, one IDC of recent onset) and they all remained stable post-explantation. The remaining two had chronic IDC and experienced a reduction of EF shortly after explantation, without clinical consequences. On the other hand, all supported patients improved their exercise tolerance and there was no discrimination of this parameter with genuine recovery. It should be noted that exercise tests were performed under maximal support. However, improvement of skeletal muscle function may act as a confounding factor for interpretation of the results of cardiopulmonary stress test in patients with LVADs.

In 2006, the Harefield group, led by Magdi Yacoub, reported the most intriguing data, as far as bridge to recovery protocols are concerned. They proposed and evaluated a combination therapy involving LVAD support to achieve maximal unloading of the myocardium, together with pharmacological therapy at the maximal tolerated doses, aiming at reversal of remodeling, followed by addition of pharmacologic stimulation of the β2 receptors by clenbuterol, for the development of physiological hypertrophy of the cardiac muscle. More specifically, ACE inhibitors, angiotensin 1 receptor antagonists, spironolactone and beta blockers with their well established effect on reverse remodeling were administered to the mechanically supported patients. Once maximal reverse remodeling had been achieved, a program of inducing physiological hypertrophy was instituted. This consisted of administration of the beta-2 agonist clenbuterol which is known to induce skeletal muscle hypertrophy (Petrou et al., 1995) and improve performance, as well as to stimulate physiological 'myocardial hypertrophy' (Wong et al., 1998). Evidence of recovery was monitored by repeated echocardiographic measurements and a '6 min walk' test with the device (pulsatile HeartMate XVE) switched off (on heparin). Patients also underwent cardiopulmonary exercise stress test, right and left heart catheterization (including left and right heart pressures, cardiac output with the device on and off, left ventricular angiography and left ventricular biopsies). Explantation was considered if the following criteria were met (with the device off for 15 minutes): a) left ventricular end-diastolic diameter < 60 mm; left ventricular end-systolic diameter <50mm; LVEF >45%; left ventricular end-diastolic pressure (or pulmonary-capillary wedge pressure) < 12 mm Hg; a resting cardiac index > 2.8 l/m^2; maximal oxygen consumption (VO2 max) with exercise > 16 ml/kg/min and a VE/VCO2 slope < 34. Explantation of the device was feasible in 73% of the patients with idiopathic dilated cardiomyopathy who could be enrolled in the study (or in 46% of all the IDC patients that underwent implantation of an LVAD at this period in their center), with 100% and 89% cumulative rates of freedom from recurrent HF at 1 and 4 years, respectively (Birks et al., 2006). It should be noted that patients who could be weaned from LVAD support, not only fulfilled the above mentioned criteria, but achieved values within the normal range on these tests: LVEF of 64±8% before explantation (12±6% before implantation, P=0.001), left ventricular end-diastolic diameter of 55.9±8.3 mm (compared with 75.1±16.3 mm, P=0.002), mean left ventricular end-systolic diameter 39.6±6.5 mm (compared with 66.9±16.3 mm, P=0.002). Before explantation, VO2 max (with the pump off) was 20.7±6.1 ml/kg/min and VE/VCO2 slope 32.5±7.9. Pulmonary-capillary wedge pressure before explantation (with the device off for 15 min) was 9.0±4.1 mm Hg and cardiac index 2.8±0.7 l/m^2. Interestingly, the same group demonstrated better results for quality of life in the bridge to recovery group 3.6 years after LVAD removal, compared to bridge to transplantation patients and even to transplanted patients (George et al., 2008). These impressive data proved that in carefully selected patients, long term, stable myocardial recovery can be achieved and this may be a legitimate treatment target for IDC patients requiring mechanical support, in order to improve not only their prognosis and quality of life but also donor organ allocation, particularly in the era of donor organ shortage. However, selecting the appropriate candidates for this treatment remains a formidable task, since there are no criteria to predict which patient will experience recovery and if this improvement is going to be sustained for a long enough period to justify the risks of withdrawing mechanical support.

Extremely important data became also available from Hetzer's group in Berlin. They were able to wean 24.4% of 131 DCM patients from LVAD support (pulsatile devices in the vast majority) (Dandel et al., 2005). They also used off-pump tests in order to obtain echocardiographic measurements. An LV diastolic diameter < 55 mm and and LVEF> 45% were considered criteria for complete recovery, however they proceeded to device explantation in some patients with evidence of partial recovery. When patients were considered for device removal, an off-pump right heart catheterization was performed and normal right atrial and capillary wedge pressures were mandatory before proceeding to explantation. Twenty two / 32 patients experienced clinical stability for at least 3 years, whereas in 10 patients heart failure recurred and 8 of them required cardiac transplantation. Partial recovery in the echocardiogram as well as a history of IDC for more than five years was predictors of heart failure recurrence.

The same investigators also reported results about long term clinical stability of 35 IDC patients successfully weaned from LVAD support (Dandel et al., 2008). Decision for LVAD explantation was made based on off-pump echocardiographic assessment. For pulsatile devices, a complete cessation of LVAD operation was induced, under full heparinization. For continuous flow devices, echocardiography was performed after reduction of pump rate (revolutions per minute) at the lowest levels where retrograde flow (from the aorta to the LV) through the device was not observed. In addition to the above mentioned criteria, geometry of the LV was also assessed and LV relative wall thickness (RWT) >0.30 and sphericity index < 0.8 were considered favorable indices. Recurrence of heart failure was observed in 16/35 of the patients and again evidence of partial recovery in the echocardiogram as well as a history of heart failure of more than 5 years and a required LV support duration of more than 6 months for induction of recovery.

Recently, the Harefield group, using the same medical treatment protocol published data from 19 patients with non ischemic cardiomyopathy, who received a continuous flow LVAD (Thoratec HeartMate II) as a bridge to recovery. LV function was monitored with monthly postimplantation echocardiographic measurements of the LV diameters and LVEF. As already mentioned, no real off-pump test can be performed with continuous flow pumps, because cessation of rotor function would result in backflow of blood from the aorta to the LV through the device, and therefore it would impose a tremendous volume overload on the LV. Therefore, the investigators performed echocardiograms, as well as 6-minute walk and cardiopulmonary exercise tests both with the device at optimal speed and after reduction of the level of support at 6000 rpm, where no regurgitation would occur. Right and left heart cardiac catheterizations were performed before explantation, again with the device at optimal speed and at 6000 rpm for at least 15 minutes. Using the same criteria for explantation as in their original study, complete recovery that allowed device explantation was achieved in 12/19 patients (63.2%), after 286±97 days. Estimated survival without heart failure recurrence was 83.3% at 1 and 3 years. Before explantation, at low flow for 15 minutes, ejection fraction was 70 ± 7%, left ventricular end-diastolic diameter was 48.6 ± 5.7 mm, left ventricular end-systolic diameter was 32.3 ± 5.7 mm, VO2peak was 21.6 ± 4 mL/kg/min, pulmonary capillary wedge pressure was 5.9 ± 4.6 mm Hg, and cardiac index was 3.6 ± 0.6 L/min/ m^2, indicating again that complete normalization of LV function and hemodynamics is associated with clinical stability and better long term outcome after explantation.

Importantly, this group thoroughly investigated methods to assess cardiac function under support with a continuous flow LVAD (Thoratec HeartMate II). They performed echocardiography at gradually lower rates of pump rotor speed and confirmed that at a fixed rate of 6000rpm, no forward or backward flow through the device could be identified. Therefore, pump speed at 6000rpm can induce physiologic loading on the LV and can be used for valid off-pump evaluations (George et al 2010). The same investigators also tried to clarify the role of optimal pump speed function on cardiopulmonary exercise stress test parameters. They were able to demonstrate that a rapid reduction of pump speed from optimal to 6000 rpm resulted in a reduction of VO2peak of 23% and of exercise duration of 18%. Despite the fact that multiple factors can influence exercise tolerance, and therefore a single value of VO2peak that can be considered threshold discriminating recovered patients probably does not exist, the relative change of this parameter between a test performed at optimal pump speed and at 6000 rpm is very important. Although this issue has never been addressed directly, ideally for a patient to be considered eligible for device explantation, these two values should not be significantly different (Jakovljevic et al., 2010).

Recently, stress echocardiography has been used in order to establish echocardiographic criteria for better evaluation of the native heart. In exercised patients, the systolic mitral annular motion increases significantly in parallel with cardiac output and the ratio of peak mitral E-wave velocity to early mitral annulus velocity (E/e'), has been demonstrated as a good approximation of LV filling pressures during exercise. These two parameters can be used as indices of cardiac output and pulmonary pressures in mechanically supported patients, even during off-pump tests.

In conclusion, although more or less similar methods are being used for LV function assessment during LVAD support, by most of the expert groups, criteria to diagnose recovery and results concerning the possibility for weaning from mechanical support vary considerably. There are no universally accepted patient selection criteria, as well as parameters that will safely predict adequate recovery and long term clinical stability after device explantation. Currently used criteria by most of the experienced groups for detection of recovery, as well as appropriate evaluation tests for pulsatile and non-pulsatile devices are summarized in Tables 1, 2 and 3.

	LVEF	LVIDd	PCWP	RAP	VO2max
Dandel et al., 2005	≥45%	≤ 55mm	≤10mmHg	≤8mmHg	-
Maybaum et al., 2007	≥40%	-	-	-	-
Mancini et al., 1998	-	≤ 55mm	≤10mmHg	-	20ml/kg/min
Yacoub et al., 2006, 2011	≥45%	≤ 60mm (LVESD<50mm)	≤12mmHg	-	>16ml/kg/min (VE/VCO2slope< 34)
Muller et al., 1997	≥41%	≤58mm	-	-	-

Table 1. Criteria for LVAD explantation, in different studies

On- pump	Off-pump
echocardiography (LVEF, LVEDD, LVESD, mitral E/A ratio, tricuspid regurgitation velocity, pulmonary valve acceleration time)	
doboutamine echocardiography (same parameters as above)	
cardiopulmonary exercise testing (VO2max, VE/VCO2slope)	
right heart catheterization (PCWP, RAP)	
6 min walking test	

Table 2. Tests used for recovery detection during support with pulsatile mechanical assist devices

Optimal speed (≈ 9000-10000rpm)	Reduced level of support (revolutions per minute: 6000rpm)
echocardiography (LVEF, LVEDD, LVESD, mitral E/A ratio, tricuspid regurgitation velocity, pulmonary valve acceleration time)	
doboutamine echocardiography (same parameters as above)	
cardiopulmonary exercise testing (VO2max, VE/VCO2slope)	
right heart catheterization (PCWP, RAP)	
6 min walking test	

Table 3. Tests used for recovery detection during support with non- pulsatile mechanical assist devices

10. Assessment of cardiac function during LVAD support as bridge to transplantation or destination therapy

Although recovery during support with an LVAD is an intriguing concept that merits further investigation, in everyday clinical practice, there are several more common reasons why native LV function should be monitored, despite the presence of an LVAD. During the recent years, data have accumulated about the long term problems that can manifest in patients supported by an LVAD, even many years after the implantation.

10.1 Determine optimal settings of LVAD function

Currently, continuous flow (axial or centrifugal) pumps are by far the most frequently used ones in the clinical practice, for long term patient support. Although maintaining adequate cardiac output to preserve end organ function and allow patients to be completely asymptomatic in their daily activities is an obvious need, optimal rotor speed of these pumps has not been determined yet, and seems to be a highly individualized parameter. For this decision, echocardiography provides the most easily accessible and valuable information. Many echocardiographic parameters should be taken into account, including LV and RV dimensions, the presence of mitral or tricuspid valve insufficiency, the shape of the interatrial or interventricular septum. At optimal pump interventricular and interatrial septum are at neutral position or slightly shifted to the left, whereas mitral and tricuspid valve regurgitation are minimal. Although, it is sometimes difficult to obtain good echocardiographic images in these patients, due to the apical cannula that often interferes with image acquisition, echocardiography remains the modality of choice for this kind of assessment, since it is noninvasive and widely available.

10.2 Aortic valve function

As far as the aortic valve is concerned, pulsed-wave Doppler can be used to assess flow across this valve. In patients with continuous flow mechanical support, aortic valve closure during the entire cardiac cycle has been found in up to 83% of patients, whereas a minority has intermittent opening with no detectable flow across the valve (Topilsky et al., 2011). This happens because at high pump speeds, the device unloads the LV at a point where LV systolic pressure is lower than aortic pressure and thus the aortic valve remains closed. On the other hand, with lowering of the revolutions per minute (RPM), the percentage of cardiac cycles where opening of the aortic valve occurs increases substantially. A continuously closed valve can have leaflet fusion as a consequence. This is commonly observed in patients with continuous flow LVADs and can have severe implications. Blood stasis and eventually thrombosis increases the risk of thromboembolic events and therefore more intense anticoagulation is needed. Aortic insuffiency can also develop or worsen (if preexisting) when the valve is constantly closed. The cause of this type of insufficiency is multifactorial; loss of pulsatility and chronically elevated aortic root pressure (the smaller device outflow diameter requires higher velocities to maintain the appropriate flow) produce high radial aortic root sheer stress, valve malcoaptation and finally aortic insufficiency. In addition, lack of regular aortic valve opening may independently promote valve thickening and fusion.

Recently it was reported that 6% of the patients with HMI will develop aortic insufficiency after a mean duration of 50 days of mechanical support and 11% after 1 year; 14% of the patients with HMII after 90 days of mechanical support and 25% after 1 year. This fact points out the importance of pre-operative evaluation of the aortic valve in order to detect valve insufficiency and address it surgically during implantation. Moreover, since HMII is being increasingly used for destination therapy, it is important to exercise vigorous postoperative surveillance of these patients for aortic insufficiency development. In this direction frequent evaluation with echocardiography of the aortic root is mandatory, since aorta often dilates during mechanical support, especially in HMII patients who have closed aortic valves. In patients who can tolerate lower pump speeds without developing symptoms or signs of low cardiac output and end organ hypoperfusion, setting device function at a level that allows aortic valve opening every 3rd to 5th cardiac circle may ameliorate the problem.

10.3 Right ventricular function

Monitoring right ventricular function not only before but also after LVAD implantation is also crucial. As already mentioned right ventricular failure develops in about 20-30% of the patients supported with an LVAD. Under normal conditions, after LVAD implantation, the unloading of the LV reduces left atrial and mean pulmonary pressure improving right ventricular function. However, abnormal interventricular septum shift towards the left during unloading of the LV reduces the efficiency of RV contraction and additionally the elevated RV preload can deteriorate even more RV function leading to RV failure, which is associated with very high post-LVAD morbidity and mortality rates. RV failure after LVAD implantation increases the perioperative mortality rate from 10%–15% for those without RV failure to 38%–43% (Matthews et al., 2008).

Preoperative evaluation of RV and intraoperative and postoperative protection of RV function and management of RV failure are beyond the scope of the present manuscript. However RV failure may develop even late after LVAD implantation, as a cause of chronically increased RV preload (due to the increased cardiac output by the LVAD and parallel increased venous return), increased wall stress, changes in geometry of the RV in case of excessive leftward shift of the intraventricular septum and progressive tricuspid annular dilatation, which results in reduced tricuspid valve coaptation and increased RV preload due to tricuspid regurgitation. It must be emphasized that the RV is diseased in most of the times (cardiomyopathy, prior right ventricular myocardial infarction) and therefore poorly tolerates chronically elevated preload. Periodical echocardiographic assessments after LVAD implantation should be performed and if RV failure is detected appropriate therapeutic measures should be applied, i.e. reduction of pump speed if possible, in order to reduce preload and avoid excessive IVS leftward shift and diuretics to decrease RV preload. The role of RV afterload reducing agents, such as sildenafil, that can selectively reduce pulmonary vascular resistance, has not been studied in this clinical setting, but in theory appears as an attractive option.

10.4 Mitral valve function

MV regurgitation is rarely a problem in LVAD patients. LV unloading during LVAD support reduces LV size and filling pressures, improves coaptation of the MV leaflets and significantly reduces MR. In case mitral regurgitation appears after continuous LVAD implantation, inadequate LV decompression should be suspected and the possibility of increasing LVAD speed should be considered. Pulsatile LVADs by operating in a full-to-empty mode reduce the mitral regurgitation more than continuous-flow LVADs.

10.5 Assessment of device function-malfunction

Since device malfunctions may appear at any time after implantation (17% of deaths in REMATCH trial), if the patient's cardiac function is known to be severely compromised, emergency device exchange may be required even before symptomatic heart failure develops. The most common cause of continuous LVAD dysfunction is impeller thrombosis, which leads to reduced LVAD flow, and increased power use by the device. In this case, left ventricle is not fully unloaded and the increase in LV end diastolic volume will cause significant functional mitral regurgitation, right sift of the interventricular and interatrium septum and opening of the aortic valve in every LV contraction. In addition to these echocardiographic findings, laboratory analysis in patients with intravascular hemolysis will reveal increased LDH, plasma hemoglobin, bilirubin and D-dimers.

11. Conclusion – Future perspectives

Although the role of left ventricular assist devices as a bridge to transplantation or destination therapy is well established and high success rates have been achieved, the active monitoring of these patients for possible recovery is desirable for many reasons. For bridge to transplant patients, shortage of donor organs mandates the best allocation possible and removal from the list even of a small number of patients would increase the chances for a transplant of those who don't have other options. For patients initially selected for destination, recovery and device explantation would relieve them from risks of device related morbidity and mortality (device malfunction, thrombosis, bleeding and infection).
In order to materialize this very ambitious target, several prerequisites need to be satisfied:

- Criteria for optimal patient selection should be developed. These will rely on accurate diagnosis of the underlying disease that led to heart failure as well as disease duration.
- Optimal pharmacologic management of bridge to recovery patients needs to be established. Drug regimen should probably include all the available anti-remodeling substances, at maximal tolerated doses, and possibly β2-stimulation, but the efficacy of this approach needs to be demonstrated in randomized trials.
- Reliable protocols for evaluation of cardiac function under mechanical support need to be applied. These should be based on some type of off-pump test, depending on device type, and involve echocardiography, right heart catheterization and exercise stress test. It is not only the presence of good function of the native left ventricle that needs to be detected, but also long term stability that needs to be predicted. The latter remains the most challenging task currently. More prolonged in duration evaluation tests (than the ones used in most of the studies until now), using operation of the pump at the lowest possible rates in terms of safety, need to be tested in future studies.
- Histological, cellular and molecular indices of genuine recovery (as opposed to simple markers of unloading) are the subject of intense research and are expected to greatly contribute to the accurate diagnosis of significant ventricular recovery during mechanical support (Drakos et al., 2007).

LVADs designed specifically for recovery (easily implantable and explantable, atraumatic to the myocardium, operating in coordination with the native heart) are currently under development and may find a place in clinical practice in the future (Nanas et al., 1996). The principal of counterpulsation appears particularly promising for this purpose, since the LV can be very effectively unloaded, while at the same time it maintains adequate function for atrophy to be prevented. In addition, using different levels of support (every cardiac cycle, or 1-2, 1-3 etc) cardiac function can be easily assessed and monitored. Implantable counterpulsation devices may be used in carefully selected candidates for recovery; if there is successful outcome, they can easily be removed, otherwise, they can serve as bridge to a permanent device implantation or transplantation.

12. References

Altieri, FD.; Watson, JT. & Taylor, KD.(1986). Mechanical support for the failing heart. *J Biomater Appl.* Vol. 1, (July 1986), pp. 106-56.

Ammar, KA.; Jacobsen, SJ. & Mahoney, DW. (2007). Prevalence and prognostic significance of heart failure stages: application of the American College of Cardiology/American Heart Association heart failure staging criteria in the community. *Circulation*, Vol. 115, (March 2007), pp.1563–1570.

Barbone, A.; Holmes, W.; Heerdt, PM.; The' AH.; Naka, Y.; Joshi, N.; Daines, M.; Marks, AR.; Oz, MC. & Burkhoff, D. (2001) Comparison of right and left ventricular responses to left ventricular assist device support in patients with severe heart failure: a primary role of mechanical unloading underlying reverse remodeling. *Circulation,* Vol. 104, (August 2001), pp. 670-5.

Bartoli, CR.; Giridharan, GA.; Litwak, KN.; Sobieski, M.; Prabhu, SD.; Slaughter, MS. & Koenig, SC. (2010) Hemodynamic responses to continuous versus pulsatile mechanical unloading of the failing left ventricle. *ASAIO J*, Vol. 56, (September 2010) , No 5, pp. 410-6.

Bashore, TM.; Magorien, DJ.; Letterio, J.; Shaffer, P. & Unverferth, DV. (1987) Histologic and biochemical correlates of left ventricular chamber dynamics in man. *JACC* , Vol. 9 , (April 1987), pp. 734-742

Birks, EJ.; Tansley, PD.; Hardy, J.; George, RS.; Bowles, CT.; Burke, M.; Banner, NR.; Khaghani, A. & Yacoub, MH.(2006) Left ventricular assist device and drug therapy for the reversal of heart failure. *N Engl J Med*, Vol. 355, (November 2006), pp. 1873–1884.

Birks, EJ.; George, RS.; Hedger, M.; Bahrami, T.; Wilton, P.; Bowles, CT.; Webb, C.; Bougard, R.; Amrani, M.; Yacoub, MH.; Dreyfus, G. & Khaghani, A. (2011) Reversal of severe heart failure with a continuous-flow left ventricular assist device and pharmacological therapy: a prospective study Circulation, Vol. 123, (February 2011), No. 4, pp. 381-90.

Burkhoff, D.; Flaherty, JT.; Yue, DT.; Herskowitz, A.; Oikawa, RY.; Sugiura, S.; Franz, MR.; Baumgartner ,WA.; Schaefer, J.; Reitz BA. & Sagawa, K. (1988). In vitro studies of isolated supported human hearts. *Heart Vessels*, Vol. 4, (1988), pp. 185-196

Curtis, LH.; Whellan, DJ.; Hammill, BG.; Hernandez, AF.; Anstrom, KJ.; Shea, AM. & Schulman, KA (2008) Incidence and prevalence of heart failure in elderly persons, 1994–2003. *Arch. Intern. Med*, Vol. 168, (February 2008), pp. 418–424.

Dandel, M.; Weng, Y.; Siniawski H.; Potapov, E.; Lehmkuhl, HB. & Hetzer, R. (2005) Long-term results in patients with idiopathic dilated cardiomyopathy after weaning from left ventricular assist devices. *Circulation*, Vol. 112(August 2005), pp. I37-45.

Dandel, M.; Weng, Y.; Siniawski, H.; Potapov, E.; Drews, T.; Lehmkuhl, HB.; Knosalla, C. & Hetzer, R. (2008) Prediction of cardiac stability after weaning from left ventricular assist devices in patients with idiopathic dilated cardiomyopathy. *Circulation*, Vol. 118, (September 2008) pp. S94-105.

DeRose, JJR.; Michael, A. & Sun, B.(1997). Implantable left ventricular assist devices: an evolving long-term cardiac replacement therapy. *Ann Surg,* Vol. 226, (October 1997), pp.461–70.

Dipla, K.; Mattiello, J.A.; Jeevanandam, V.; Houser, S.R. & Margulies, K.B. (1998) Myocyte recovery after mechanical circulatory support in humans with end-stage heart failure. *Circulation,* Vol. 97, (June 1998), pp. 2316–2322.

Drakos SG.; Terrovitis JV.; Anastasiou-Nana MI. & Nanas JN. (2007) Reverse remodeling during long-term mechanical unloading of the left ventricle. *J Mol Cell Cardiol.*, Vol. 43, (September 2007) pp. 231-42.

El-Banayosy, A.; Arusoglu, L.& Kizner, L. (2000) Novacor left ventricular assist systems versus HeartMate vented electric left ventricular system as a long mechanical support device in bridging patients: a prospective study. *J Thoracic Cardiovasc Surg,* Vol. 119, (March 2000), pp.581–587.

El-Banayosy, A.; Arusoglu, L.; Kizner, L.; Fey, O.; Sarnowski, P.; Morshuis, M.; Milting, H.; Koertke, H. & Koerfer, R. 2001. Hemodynamic exercise testing reveals a low incidence of myocardial recovery in LVAD patients. (2001) *J. Heart Lung Transplant,* Vol. 20, (February 2001) pp. 209–210.

Farrar, D.J.; Holman, W.R.; McBride, L.R.; Kormos, R.L.; Icenogle, T.B.; Hendry, P.J.; Moore, C.H.; Loisance, D.Y.; El-Banayosy, A. & Frazier, H. (2002). Long-term follow-up of thoratec ventricular assist device bridge-to-recovery patients successfully removed from support after recovery of ventricular function. *J. Heart Lung Transplant,* Vol. 21, (May 2002), pp. 516–521.

Frazier, OH.; Benedict, CR.; Radovancevic, B.; Bick, RJ.; Capek, P.; Springer, WE.; Macris, MP.; Delgado, R. & Buja, LM. (1996). Improved left ventricular function after chronic left ventricular unloading. *Ann Thorac Surg,* Vol. 62, (September 1996), No 3, pp.675-81.

George, RS.; Yacoub, MH.; Bowles, CT.; Hipkin, M.; Rogers, P.; Hallas, C.; Banner, NR.; Dreyfus, G.; Khaghani, A. & Birks, EJ.(2008) Quality of life after removal of left ventricular assist device for myocardial recovery. *J Heart Lung Transplant,* Vol. 27, (February 2008), No. 2, pp. 165-72.

George, RS.; Sabharwal, NK.; Webb, C.; Yacoub, MH.; Bowles, CT.; Hedger, M.; Khaghani, A. & Birks EJ (2010) Echocardiographic assessment of flow across continuous-flow ventricular assist devices at low speeds. *J Heart Lung Transplant.* (November 2010), Vol.29, pp.1245-52.

Givertz, MM. & Colucci, WS. (1998). New targets for heart-failure therapy: endothelin, inflammatory cytokines, and oxidative stress. *Lancet,* Vol. 352, (August 1998), pp. SI34-SI38.

Grinda, J.M.; Chevalier, P.; D'Attellis, N.; Bricourt, M.O.; Berrebi, A.; Guibourt, P.; Fabiani, J.N. & Deloche, A. (2004) Fulminant myocarditis in adults and children: bi-ventricular assist device for recovery. *Eur. J. Cardiothorac. Surg,* Vol. 26, (December 2004) pp. 1169–1173.

Hall, S.; Cigarroa, C.; Marcouz, L.; Hatfield, B.; Peters, A.; Grayburn, PA. & Eichhorn, EJ. (1994). Regression of hypertrophy and alteration in left ventricular geometry in patients with congestive heart failure treated with beta-adrenergic blockade. *Circulation,* Vol. 90, (1994), pp. 543.

Helman, D.N.; Maybaum, S.W.; Morales, D.L.; Williams, M.R.; Beniaminovitz, A.; Edwards, N.M.; Mancini, D.M. & Oz, M.C. (2000) Recurrent remodeling after ventricular assistance: is long-term myocardial recovery attainable? *Ann. Thorac. Surg*, Vol. 70, (October 2000), pp. 1255–1258.

Hogness, JR (1991)*The artificial heart*, National Academy Press, Washington.

Hon JK. & Yacoub MH (2003) Bridge to recovery with the use of left ventricular assist device and clenbuterol. *Ann Thorac Surg,*, Vol. 75, (June 2003), pp. S36-41.

Jakovljevic, DG.; George, RS.; Nunan, D.; Donovan, G.; Bougard, RS.; Yacoub, MH.; Birks, EJ. & Brodie DA (2010) The impact of acute reduction of continuous-flow left ventricular assist device support on cardiac and exercise performance. *Heart*, (September 2010), Vol. 96, pp.1390-5.

Josue, O.(1907) Hypertrophie cardioque caus'ee par l'adrenaline et la toxine typhique. *C R Soc Biol*, Vol. 63, (1907), pp.285–290.

Jugdutt, BL. & Warnica, JW. (1988). Intravenous nitroglycerin therapy to limit myocardial infarct size, expansion and complications: effect of timing, dosage and infarct location.(1988). *Circulation*, Vol.78, (October 1988), pp.906-919.

Katz, AM (1988) Cellular mechanisms in congestive heart failure. *Am J Cardiol* , Vol. 11, No. 62, (July 1988), pp. 3A-8A

Klotz, S.; Deng, MC.; Stypmann, J.; Roetker, J.; Wilhelm, MJ. & Hammel, D.(2004). Left ventricular pressure and volume unloading during pulsatile versus nonpulsatile left ventricular assist device support. *Ann Thorac Surg*, Vol. 77, (January 2004), pp.143–9.

Klotz, S.; Naka, Y.; Oz, M.C. & Burkhoff, D. (2005) Biventricular assist device-induced right ventricular reverse structural and functional remodeling. *J. Heart Lung Transplant*, Vol. 24, (September 2005), pp. 1195–1201

Lahpor JR (2009) State of the art: implantable ventricular assist devices. Curr Opin Organ Transplant Vol.14, (October 2009), pp. 554-9.

LeGrice, IJ.; Takayama, Y.; Holmes, JW. & Covell, JW. (1995). Impaired subendocardial function in tachycardia-induced cardiac failure. *Am J Physiol*, Vol. 268, (May 1995), pp. H1788–H1794.

Levin, HR.; Chen, JM.; Oz, MC.; Catanese, KA.; Krum, H.; Goldsmith, RL.; Packer, M. & Rose, EA. (1994) Potential of left ventricular assist devices as outpatient therapy while awaiting transplantation. *Ann Thorac Surg*, Vol. 58, (November 1994), No. 5, pp. 1515-20.

Levin, HR.; Oz, MC.; Chen, JM.; Packer, M.; Rose, EA. & Burkhoff, D. (1995) Reversal of Chronic Ventricular Dilation in Patients With End-Stage Cardiomyopathy by Prolonged Mechanical Unloading. *Circulation*, Vol. 91 (June 1995), pp. 2717-2720.

Levin, HR.; Oz, MC.; Catanese, KA.; Rose, EA. & Burkhoff, D.(1996) Transient normalization of systolic and diastolic function after support with a left ventricular assist device in a patient with dilated cardiomyopathy. *J Heart Lung Transplant*, Vol. 15, (August 1996), pp. 840-2.

Levine, TB. & Levine AB. (1990) Regional blood flow supply and demand in heart failure. Am Heart J. Vol. 120, (December 1990), pp.1547-51.

Levy, D.; Kenchaiah, S.; Larson, MG.; Benjamin, EJ.; Kupka, MJ.; Ho, KK.; Murabito, JM. & Vasan, RS. (2002). Long-term trends in the incidence of and survival with heart failure. *N. Engl. J. Med*, Vol. 347, (October 2002), pp. 1397–1402.

Li YY.; Feldman AM.; Sun Y. & McTiernan CF. Differential expression of tissue inhibitors of metalloproteinases in the failing human heart (1998) *Circulation,* Vol.98, (October 1998), pp. 1728 -1734.

Lloyd-Jones, D.M.; Larson, MG.; Leip, EP.; Beiser, A.; D'Agostino, RB.; Kannel, WB.; Murabito, JM.; Vasan ,RS.; Benjamin, EJ. & Levy, D.(2002). Lifetime risk for developing congestive heart failure: the Framingham Heart Study. *Circulation,* (December 2002), Vol. 106, pp. 3068–3072.

Lloyd-Jones, D. (2010). Heart disease and stroke statistics—2010 update: a report from the American Heart Association. *Circulation,* Vol. 121, (March 2010), pp. 46–215

Madigan, JD.; Barbone, A.; Choudhri, AF.; Morales, DLS.; Cai, B.; Oz, MC. & Burkhoff, D. (2001) Time course of reverse remodeling of the left ventricle during support with a left ventricular assist device. *J Thorac Cardiovasc Surg,* Vol. 121, (May 2001), pp. 902–8.

Mancini, D.M.; Beniaminovitz, A.; Levin, H.; Catanese, K.; Flannery, M.; DiTullio, M.; Savin, S.; Cordisco, M.E.; Rose, E. & Oz, M.; (1998). Low incidence of myocardial recovery after left ventricular assist device implantation in patients with chronic heart failure. *Circulation,* Vol. 98, (December 1998), pp. 2383–2389.

Mann, DL.; Kent, RL.; Parsons, B. & Cooper, G IV. (1992) Adrenergic effects on the biology of the adult mammalian cardiocyte. *Circulation,* Vol. 85, (February 1992), pp. 790–804.

Marx, S.O.; Reiken, S.; Hisamatsu, Y.; Jayaraman, T.; Burkhoff, D.; Rosemblit, N. & Marks, A.R. (2000). PKA phosphorylation dissociates FKBP12.6 from the calcium release channel (ryanodine receptor): defective regulation in failing hearts. *Cell,* Vol. 101, (May 2001), pp. 365–376.

Matthews, JC.; Koelling, TM.; Pagani, FD. & Aaronson KD(2008) The right ventricular failure risk score a pre-operative tool for assessing the risk of right ventricular failure in left ventricular assist device candidates. *J Am Coll Cardiol,* Vol. 51, (June 2008), pp.2163–2172.

Maybaum, S.; Mancini, D.; Xydas, S.; Starling, RC.; Aaronson, K.; Pagani, FD.; Miller, LW.; Margulies, K.; McRee, S.; Frazier, OH. & Torre-Amione, G.; LVAD Working Group. (2007) Cardiac Improvement During Mechanical Circulatory Support: A Prospective Multicenter Study of the LVAD Working Group. *Circulation,* Vol. 115, (May 2007), pp. 2497-2505

McCarthy, PM.; Savage, RM.; Fraser, CD.; Vargo, R.; James, KB. & Goormastic, M. (1995). Hemodynamic and physiologic changes during support with an implantable left ventricular assist device. *J Thorac Cardiovasc Surg* , Vol. 109, (March 1995), pp.409–17

McCarthy, PM.; Smedira, NO.; Vargo, RL.; Goormastic, M.; Hobbs, RE.; Starling, RC. & Young, JB. (1998). One hundred patients with the HeartMate left ventricular assist device: evolving concepts and technology. *J Thorac Cardiovasc Surg.*, Vol. 115, (April 1998), No 4, pp :904-12.

Miller LW.; Pagani FD.; Russell SD.; John R.; Boyle AJ.; Aaronson KD.; Conte JV.; Naka Y.; Mancini D.;, Delgado RM.; MacGillivray TE.; Farrar DJ. & Frazier OH. (2007). Use of a continuous-flow device in patients awaiting heart transplantation. *N Engl J Med,* Vol. 357, (August 2007), pp. 885-896.

Müller, J.; Wallukat, G.; Weng, YG.; Dandel, M.; Spiegelsberger, S.; Semrau, S.; Brandes, K.; Theodoridis, V.; Loebe, M.; Meyer, R. & Hetzer, R. (1997) Weaning from mechanical cardiac support in patients with idiopathic dilated cardiomyopathy. *Circulation,* Vol. 96, (July 1997), No. 2, pp. 542-9.

Nanas, J.; Lolas, CT.; Charitos, CE.; Nanas, SN.; Margari, ZJ.; Agapitos, EV.; Moulopoulos, SD. (1996). A valveless high stroke volume counterpulsation device restores hemodynamics in patients with congestive heart failure and intractable cardiogenic shock awaiting heart transplantation. *J Thorac Cardiovasc Surg, Vol.* 111, (September 1996), pp.55-61.

Ochiai, Y.; McCarthy, P.M.; Smedira, N.G.; Banbury, M.K.; Navia, J.L.; Feng, J.; Hsu, A.P.; Yeager, M.L.; Buda, T.; Hoercher, K.J.; Howard, M.W.; Takagaki, M.; Doi, K. & Fukamachi, K. (2002). Predictors of severe right ventricular failure after implantable left ventricular assist device insertion: analysis of 245 patients. *Circulation*, Vol. 106, (September 2002), pp. I198–I202.

Petrou, M.; Wynne, DG.; Boheler, KR.; Yacoub, MH. (1995) Clenbuterol induces hypertrophy of the latimus dorsi muscle and heart in the rat with molecular and phenotypic changes. *Circulation*, Vol. 92, (November 1995), pp. II-483–II-489.

Pfeffer, MA.; Lamas, G.; Vaughan, D.; Parisi, A. & Braunwald, E. (1988). Effect of captopril on progressive ventricular dilation after anterior myocardial infarction. *N Engl J Med*, Vol. 319, (July 1988), pp.80-86.

Shannon, RP.; Komamura, K.; Shen, YT.; Bishop, SP. & Vatner, SF .(1993) Impaired regional subendocardial coronary flow reserve in conscious dogs with pacing-induced heart failure.. *Am J Physiol*, Vol. 265, (September 1993), pp. H801–H809.

Simon, MA.; Kormos, RL.; Murali, S.; Nair, P.; Heffernan, M.; Gorcsan, J.; Winowich, S. & McNamara, DM. (2005) Myocardial recovery using ventricular assist devices: prevalence, clinical characteristics, and outcomes. *Circulation*. Vol. 112, (August 2005), pp. I32-6.

Slaughter, MS.; Rogers, JG.; Milano, CA.; Russell,SD.; Conte, JV.; Feldman, D.; Sun B.; Tatooles, AJ.; Delgado, RM.; Long, JW.; Wozniak, TC.; Ghumman, W.; Farrar, DJ. & Frazier, OH.(2009) Advanced heart failure treated with continuous-flow left ventricular assist device. *N Engl J Med*, Vol. 361, (December 2009), pp. 2241-2251.

Stevenson, LW. & Rose EA.(2003) Left ventricular assist devices: bridges to transplantation, recovery, and destination for whom? *Circulation*, Vol. 108, (December 2003), pp. 3059-3063.

Strüber, M.; Sander, K.; Lahpor, J.; Ahn, H.; Litzler, PY.; Drakos, SG.; Musumeci, F.; Schlensak, C.; Friedrich, I.; Gustafsson , R.; Oertel, F. & Leprince, P (2008) HeartMate II left ventricular assist device:early European experience. *Eur J Card Surg* , Vol. 34, (August 2008), pp. 289–294.

Taylor, DO.; Stehlik, J. & Edwards, LB. (2009) Registry of the International Society for Heart and Lung Transplantation: Twenty sixth Official Adult Heart Transplant Report-2009. *J Heart Lung Transplant* Vol. 28, (October 2009), pp. 1007–1022.

Thohan, V.; Stetson, SJ.; Nagueh, SF.; Rivas-Gotz, C.; Koerner, MM.; Lafuente, JA.; Loebe, M.; Noon, GP. & Torre-Amione, G. (2005) Cellular and hemodynamics responses of failing myocardium to continuous flow mechanical circulatory support using the DeBakey-Noon left ventricular assist device: a comparative analysis with pulsatile-type devices. *J Heart Lung Transplant*, Vol. 24, (May 2005), No 5, pp.566-75.

Thomas, CV.; Coker, ML.; Zellner, JL.; Handy, JR.; Crumbley, JA. & Spinale, FG.(1998) Increased matrix metalloproteinase activity and selective upregulation in LV myocardium from patients with end-stage heart failure. *Circulation*, Vol. 97, (May 1998), pp. 1708 -1715.

Thoratec: Thoratec Announces Filing of PMA Seeking Destination Therapy Approval for HeartMate II. [Press release]. 2009

Topilsky, Y.; Oh, JK.; Atchison, FW.; Shah, DK.; Bichara, VM.; Schirger, JA.; Kushwaha, SS.; Pereira, NL. & Park SJ.(2011) Echocardiographic findings in stable outpatients with properly functioning HeartMate II left ventricular assist devices. *J Am Soc Echocardiogr*, Vol. 24, (February 2011), pp.157-69.

Tyagi, SC.; Kumar, S.; Voelker, DJ.; Reddy, HK.; Janicki, JS. & Curtis, JJ. (1996a) Differential gene expression of extracellular matrix components in dilated cardiomyopathy. *J Cell Biochem.*, Vol. 63, (November 1996a) pp. 185–198.

Tyagi, SC.; Campbell, SE.; Reddy, HK.; Tjahja, E. & Voelker, DJ. (1996b) Matrix metalloproteinase activity expression in infarcted, noninfarcted and dilated cardiomyopathic human hearts. *Mol Cell Biochem.*, Vol. 155, (November 1996b), pp. 13–21.

Vatner, SF.(1988) Reduced subendocardial myocardial perfusion as one mechanism for congestive heart failure. *Am J Cardiol*, Vol. 62, (September 1988), pp. 94E–98E.

Wong, K.; Boheler, KR.; Bishop, J.; Petrou, M. & Yacoub, MH. (1998) Clenbuterol induces cardiac hypertrophy with normal functional, morphological and molecular features. *Cardiovasc Research*, Vol. 37, (January 1998), pp. 115–22.

Part 2

Clinical Aspects of Ventricular Assist Devices

4

Ventricular Assist Device: Emerging Modality for Long Term Cardiac Support

Rachit Shah, Sharath Kommu,
Rohit Bhuriya and Rohit Arora
Rosalind Franklin University/ Chicago Medical School
USA

1. Introduction

More than 5 million people carry the diagnosis of heart failure in USA and almost 300,000 people die of heart failure each year in USA[1]. Heart failure remains the most common discharge diagnosis for patients older than 65 years of age. In the Western world, most heart failure is related to coronary disease, and although the survival of patients post acute myocardial infarction has improved, this has resulted in an increase in the number of patients ultimately developing heart failure[2]. Advances in medical therapy have resulted in improved survival in patients with moderate and severe heart failure, but the prognosis for end-stage heart failure patients remains poor[3-5]. In patients with end-stage heart failure cardiac transplantation remains the gold standard of cardiac replacement therapy and it has shown the greatest survival benefit. However, the supply of donor hearts is limited. There is also an increase in the number of heart failure patients who are not candidates for cardiac transplantation, mainly due to older age and presence of co-morbidities. There has therefore been considerable interest in alternative forms of cardiac replacement therapy, either as a temporary bridge to transplantation or as a definitive destination strategy. Multiple different mechanical devices for long-term circulatory support have been developed, ranging from total artificial hearts to ventricular assist devices (VADs). The main purpose of a VAD is to unload the failing heart and help maintain forward cardiac output and vital organ perfusion. Originally introduced as a temporary bridge to recovery and then as a bridge to transplantation, VADs have evolved into permanent or "destination" therapy for a growing number of patients with refractory heart failure[6].

2. History and evolution of VADs

Mechanical circulatory support is rapidly emerging as an adjunct/alternative to cardiac transplantation. Its development commenced at the National Institutes of Health in 1964 in USA with the initial focus on development of a total artificial heart, but, with few exceptions, this has had limited success[7]. The major attention has now shifted to mechanical ventricular assist devices. The first successful cardiac-assist device in humans was implanted by DeBakey at the Texas Heart Institute in 1966[78]. Early devices were large and cumbersome with extracorporeal placement and provided temporary support only. The technological advancements led to the development of pulsatile LVAD design pioneered in

1976 as the Axio-symmetrical and Pierce-Donachy LVADs. A refined version of the latter device known as the Heartmate (Thoratec) was approved by the FDA as a bridging device to cardiac transplantation in 1994[78]. Its updated version, the Heartmate XVE was approved as bridge therapy in 1998. The Randomized Evaluation of Mechanical Assistance in Treatment of Chronic Heart Failure (REMATCH) study evaluated the long term benefit of Heartmate XVE placement compared with optimal medical therapy in end-stage heart failure patients[4]. There was 48% reduction in death from all causes, attributable to LVAD therapy compared with best medical therapy in this trial. On this basis, the Heartmate XVE was approved for use as destination therapy in 2002. With time VADs have evolved significantly, with three major changes to date: (*a*) Transition from pulsatile to continuous-flow devices; (*b*) Reduction in size with the preference for internal placement of the devices; (*c*) Use of electricity as a power source[79]. The newest continuous-flow VADs are much smaller in size and are silent in operation, leading to significantly greater patient satisfaction[79]. It makes this therapy more favourable for long-term support.

3. Components of a VAD

VADs support the failing heart by unloading the ventricle and generating flow to the systemic and/or pulmonary circulation. They can be used to support the left ventricle, right ventricle or both the ventricles. LVAD (Left Ventricular Assist Device) is the main assist device used in clinical practice. Use of isolated right ventricular assist device (RVAD) is a rare event[80]. It is usually inserted around the time of placement of a (LVAD) to provide biventricular assistance. Sometimes biventricular mechanical ventricular assist devices are also used primarily for cardiac support. In comparison to single chamber VAD, biventricular mechanical devices create a complex system with two independent pumps, one right sided and the other left sided which supports both left and right ventricles.

VAD typically has an inflow cannula, an outflow cannula, a pumping chamber, per-cutaneous driveline, a controller and power supply. VADs are usually implanted through a median sternotomy, typically during cardiopulmonary bypass[80]. The inflow cannula is connected to the heart and it decompresses the ventricular cavity and an outflow cannula returns blood to either the ascending aorta or the main pulmonary artery. The pumping chamber of the VAD is implanted sub-diaphragmatically to a pre-peritoneal or intra-abdominal position or may be situated in a para-corporeal position outside the body[80]. Smaller devices are being developed for thoracic implantation, some with outflow to the descending aorta. A percutaneous driveline, containing the control and power wires, is tunnelled through the skin of the abdominal wall. It connects the device to an external portable driver consisting of an electronic or pneumatic controller and a power supply that may be worn around the waist, carried in a shoulder bag, or contained within a small bedside monitor.

Newer per-cutaneous VADs have a venous trans-septal inflow cannula that has a curved design at its end to facilitate ideal tip placement in the left atrium and contains a large end hole at its distal tip and 14 side holes to aspirate oxygenated blood from the left atrium. The cannula is attached to a continuous flow centrifugal blood pump, which in turn is driven by a 3-phase, brushless, direct current servomotor that is capable of delivering up to 5.0 L/min of blood flow. Blood is delivered from the pump to the femoral artery with an arterial perfusion catheter. This catheter ranges from 15F to17F and pumps blood from the left atrium to the right femoral artery. Alternatively, two 12F arterial perfusion catheters pump blood into the right and left femoral arteries. The pump is driven by an external microprocessor- based controller. A pressure transducer monitors the infusion pressure and identifies any disruption in the infusion line. An in-line air bubble detector monitors for the presence of air in the infusion line.

4. Types of VADs

Many VADs are currently available commercially or in various stages of development. These were developed to satisfy special needs for either short or longer-term support and, therefore, differ markedly in their design characteristics, principles of operation, hemodynamic capabilities, method of insertion, and, importantly, durability.

4.1 Percutaneous short-term devices

Percutaneous short-term VADs include devices that are inserted through the femoral artery and advanced to the left ventricle. Examples of such percutaneous short-term VADs are Impella 2.5 pump and TandemHeart. Impella 2.5 pump (Abiomed Inc., Danvers, MA) is an impeller-driven, axial flow pump, capable of pumping 2.5 L/min.[13] TandemHeart (CardiacAssist, Inc., Pittsburgh, PA) is a low speed centrifugal continuous-flow pump that drains oxygenated blood through a catheter advanced across the interatrial septum to the left atrium and pumps it back to one or both femoral arteries.[14] The experience with these devices is increasing, particularly with the Impella pump.[15,16]

4.2 Longer-term assist devices

The currently available longer-term VADs are categorized into three generations, reflecting the order in which they were developed and the type of pumping mechanism they use.

4.3 First-generation VADs

These are pulsatile devices that use pusher plates and have inflow and outflow valves. These devices are efficacious at unloading the left ventricle and maintaining the circulation, with the capacity to pump up to 10 L/min[79]. Examples of such devices are the HeartMate® I or XVE (Thoratec Corp., Pleasanton, CA) and the Novacor VAD (WorldHeart Inc., Oakland, California, USA)[81]. These implantable VADs are placed intra-abdominally or pre-peritoneally in a pocket under the abdominal rectus muscle and connected to the apex of the left ventricle and to the ascending aorta[81]. There is increased risk of hematomas and infections as they are large in volume, requiring extensive surgical dissection[81]. The percutaneous leads of these devices, especially those of the HeartMate XVE, are large and stiff and contain an air vent channel, which makes the system quite noisy and uncomfortable. All pulsatile devices have biological or mechanical valves to allow a unidirectional blood flow. Anticoagulation is necessary for all devices, except the HeartMate XVE. The latter has a textured inner surface of the pump stimulating formation of a biological layer preventing thrombus formation. Only aspirin is given as antithrombotic prophylaxis[81].

Outcomes of first-generation devices

After the REMATCH study, Heartmate XVE was approved for use as "destination therapy" (DT) in 2002. Although the VAD therapy group had significantly greater survival and quality of life at both one and two years of follow-up, the survival at two years was only 28%. In addition, there were large numbers of readmissions and device-related complications including sepsis and stroke. Therefore, use of Heartmate XVE as destination has not been widely accepted.

The first generation devices are also used successfully as a "bridge to transplantation" (BTT) with a perioperative mortality of 15-20% and an overall survival until device explantation of 60-70%[81]. However, in the majority of studies, the maximal support duration does not exceed 6 months, and in most studies mean support duration ranges only from 50 to 60 days.[17-19] Results in experienced high volume centers (>10 implants per year) tend to be better than in low-volume centers. Survival and quality of life has been closely related to adverse events such as bleeding, infections, thrombo-embolic events and technical failures. Thrombo-embolic events resulting in transient ischemic attacks or even stroke is a devastating complication. In literature, there is a high variability in rates ranging from 5 to 50%, depending on the different LVAD types and variation in anticoagulation protocols[81].

4.4 Second generation VADs

There is a need of more reliable and smaller devices due to growing waiting lists and long waiting times for heart transplantation. Second generation VADs can answer this need with smaller size and longer durability in comparison to first generation devices. The most common second generation VADs are the HeartMate 2 VAD (Thoratec Inc.), the Jarvik 2000 (Jarvik Heart Inc., New York, New York), Micromed Debakey VAD and the Berlin Heart Incor (Berlin Heart AG). They have the continuous flow impeller pumps which are considerably smaller and safer to insert. Because they have only one moving part (the rotor), they are expected to be more durable than first-generation devices. To maintain an international normalized ratio (INR) of 2.0-2.5, the use of these pumps requires full anticoagulant therapy coupled with antiplatelet medications, such as aspirin or clopidogrel. The HeartMate 2 is the most successful second-generation device with over 2500 implants worldwide. It is one-seventh of the size and one-fourth the weight of the HeartMate XVE[81].

Outcomes of second-generation devices

Heartmate II device has been approved by the US FDA for implantation as BTT in April 2008 and as DT in January 2010. The mean duration of support reported from the use of these continuous flow, rotary pumps is considerably longer compared with the first-generation devices (166–236 vs. 50–60 days). Two studies have shown 2 years survival of 65 and 69% with no mechanical failure and low fatal adverse event rates. The incidence of thrombo-embolic events in HeartMate 2 patients is in most studies comparable with those seen with Heart- Mate XVE, however the risk of hemorrhagic stroke rates tend to be higher (2-3%), probably as a result of the anticoagulation[81].

4.5 Third generation VADs

Third-generation VADs are small centrifugal pumps in which the rotor is magnetically or mechanically suspended and, therefore, does not use ball bearings. Drivelines are less thick and more flexible. These features, coupled with the lower number of revolutions per minute, should enhance durability in comparison with the second generation pumps. Examples of such third generation VADs are the VentrAssist VAD (Ventracor Ltd, Chatswood, New South Wales, Australia)[20] and the DuraHeart (Terumo, Somerset, New Jersey, USA).[21]

Outcomes of third-generation devices

These devices are thought to last as long as 5-10 years, and their performance is being evaluated in several phase I studies involving the HVAD® (Heart- Ware, Miramar, FL) devices, and more recently the DuraHeart® (Terumo Kabushiki Kaisha, Tokyo, Japan) system. They still carry the risk of neurological complications like stroke as well as risk of infections.

5. Clinical indications for VADs

Mechanical devices can be used for a wide spectrum of diseases based on the therapeutic goals of circulatory support as well as the duration of treatment. They can be used for short term as well long term duration. The indications are typically divided into 3 categories: bridge to recovery, bridge to transplantation, and destination therapy.

5.1 Bridge to recovery

VADs as a "Bridge to recovery" are used for patients who need only temporary support for days to weeks in anticipation of recovery of ventricular function followed by weaning and removal of device. This includes patients with acute inflammatory cardiomyopathies, acute cardiogenic or post-cardiotomy shock and myocardial infarction. The ability of LVADs to support an acutely failing heart while it recovers function is well documented.[16,17,33] There are observations regarding the potential for myocardial recovery even in patients with chronic heart failure.

Various studies have documented that the unloaded left ventricle undergoes a process of reverse remodeling, as categorized by multiple different indices e.g. decrease in left ventricular size[34] and normalization of pressure–volume relationship curves.[35] Cellular structure and function also improves and reverts back toward normal.[36-39] Thus, the reduction in left ventricular volumes is not just a function of the unloading provided by the VAD but actually reflects alterations in the dynamics of myocyte function.

5.2 Molecular changes in myocardium after VAD implantation

A reduction in myocardial contractility is one of the most important causes of dysfunction in heart failure.[25] Both the electrical and mechanical components of the process of excitation-contraction (E-C) coupling are altered, and Ca_2^+ handling is clearly a target for therapy in heart failure.[25] VAD therapy strongly affects E-C coupling. After VAD treatment, cardiomyocyte contractility is increased[26,27] and the force-frequency relationship is normalized.[28,29] Action-potential duration is reduced,[30,31] mirroring the shortening of the QT interval on electrocardiogram in patients after prolonged support.[32] In addition to E-C coupling mechanisms, several other molecular mechanisms responsible for VAD-induced reverse remodeling have been described. These include effects at the levels of metabolic pathways, immune and inflammatory responses, transcription factors, the adrenergic system, cytoskeletal proteins, the extracellular matrix, neurohormonal activation, and apoptosis and necrosis signaling, a breadth that suggests profound reverse remodeling at the molecular level. Clinically these changes improve left ventricular function and patients have a dramatic increase in their exercise capacity following LVAD implantation.[44-46] These findings encouraged the explantation of LVADs in select patients who have demonstrated sufficient recovery of myocardial function. To date clinical results are mixed and although the large number of studies report regression or normalization of the pathological substrate following VAD treatment, the clinical evidence for recovery remains limited. To date, an average of only 5%–10% of patients who undergo mechanical circulatory support demonstrate adequate recovery of ventricular function to allow device explantation.[33,34]

There is also concern that prolonged mechanical unloading reduces cardiac cell function, as well as cell size, in a time-dependent manner[35-40] which may lead to myocardial atrophy. Unloading induced atrophy can be an important impediment to myocardial recovery and removal of the VADs for bridge-to-recovery, limiting the efficacy of VAD treatment.[41] Minimizing unloading-induced atrophy may be an important strategy to obtain the beneficial effects of VADs and, to this end, a pharmacological regimen that includes clenbuterol has been tested in combination with VAD treatment. Clenbuterol is a unique $\beta 2$ adrenoceptor agonist that is currently approved only for patients with asthma, but has been shown in animal models to lead to significant hypertrophy of skeletal and cardiac muscle and enhanced mechanical strength of contraction.[42] A novel combination regimen including the use of five oral medications known to provide various degrees of reverse remodeling, plus clenbuterol, was used in patients with non-ischemic cardiomyopathy who were transplant candidates and required a VAD for refractory heart failure.[43] In nearly 70% of patients on the combination therapy, the VAD could be removed within one year. After four years of follow-up, the average ejection fraction had improved from 15% preoperatively to 62%. These encouraging data have prompted the initiation of the Harefield Recovery Protocol Study (HARPS). The trial will not only assess clinical cardiac recovery but also explore molecular mechanisms of clenbuterol.

5.3 Bridge to transplantation

"Bridge-to-transplantation" is the strategy in which VADs are used for improving ventricular function and peripheral perfusion in patients awaiting cardiac transplantation. Several studies have demonstrated that VADs ensure sustained improvement in hemodynamic status and quality of life in patients awaiting cardiac transplantation.[9] More than 80% of VAD-treated patients undergoing cardiac transplantation have a normal or improved post-transplant outcome.[10]

When implanted in patients refractory to medical therapy, LVADs lead to improved end organ function as well as overall physical conditioning.[10,11] LVAD markedly decreases the filling pressures and increases cardiac output by taking over the work of the left ventricle, the. This leads to lower pulmonary vascular resistance and a reduction in afterload for the right ventricle. Additionally, the increase in cardiac output provides additional preload for the right ventricle, which further enhances its function. This improvement in right ventricular function and mechanical replacement of left ventricular output by LVAD results in more efficient delivery of oxygen to end-organ tissues. As a result, the presence of the LVAD can partially or totally reverse functional impairment of these organs. This is most clearly evident in the kidneys, in which renal failure can improve or resolve following the implantation of an LVAD. All organ systems benefit from the increase in perfusion, allowing sick patients to stabilize or improve as they wait for a heart transplant. In addition to providing an increased length of time on the organ waiting list, LVADs significantly improve outcomes by reducing patients' comorbidities at the time of transplant. This makes them better transplant candidates and improves their posttransplant outcomes.[12,13]

The following criteria should generally be met prior to consideration of LVAD implant: clinical evidence of impaired end-organ perfusion with cardiac index <2 L/min/m2, pulmonary capillary wedge pressure >20 mmHg, and systolic blood pressure <80 mmHg despite maximal medical support, including inotropes and an intraaortic balloon pump, if indicated.[20] Although it is important to meet these criteria, LVAD implantation should be performed before extensive end-organ damage for maximal chance of success.[21]

5.4 Destination therapy

"Destination Therapy" is perhaps the most exciting strategy in which VADs are used as an alternative to cardiac transplant to support the patients for their entire life. It involves the largest population of the patients with end stage heart failure who are unable to receive cardiac transplantation. The success of LVAD implantation as "Bridge to transplantation" (BTT) in candidates with refractory heart failure led to the investigations for its use as an alternative to Heart transplantation HT. The first DT feasibility trials were designed over 15 years ago. The REMATCH trial was one of the most remarkable endeavours in the history of VADs that assessed the feasibility of LADs for Destination Therapy (DT). The trial was conducted between May 1998 and July 2001 at 20 US hospitals. *REMATCH trial showed significant improvement of the quality of life in patients supported with LVAD and improved one-year survival from 25% to 52%.*[4] *These data led to the US Food and Drug Administration (FDA) approval of the modified HeartMate XVE LVAD for use as DT in November 2002, thus launching a new era of surgical therapy for advanced heart failure.* One of the more recent trials the Heartmate II trial was conducted between March 2005 and May 2007 and it has shown that patients supported with HM II VAD (continuous flow VAD) had significantly improved two-year survival when compared to HM XVE recipients (58% vs. 24%, respectively) and significantly improved probability of freedom from stroke and device failure at two years, as compared to the recipients of pulsatile devices. These data led to approval of Heartmate II VAD for DT by US FDA in January 2010.

5.5 Indications for DT[82]

The criteria for VAD implantation for DT are based largely on the entry criteria into the REMATCH trial. They are:

1. Class IV NYHA symptoms for at least 60 of the last 90 days despite maximized oral therapy, including dietary salt restriction, diuretics, digitalis, beta-blockers, and angiotensin converting enzyme (ACE) inhibitors (if tolerated), or requirement of inotropic support as outlined by the AHA/ACC guidelines for heart failure treatment
2. LVEF of ≤25%,
3. Peak oxygen consumption of <12 mL/kg/min or documented inability to wean intravenous inotropic therapy owing to symptomatic hypotension, decreasing renal function, or worsening pulmonary congestion
4. Contraindication to HT due to either age greater than 65 years or comorbidities such as insulin-dependent diabetes mellitus with end-organ damage, chronic renal failure, or others, and
5. Appropriate body size (≥1.5 m2) to support the HM XVE LVAD implantation.

5.6 Survival with DT

As mentioned earlier the results of the REMATCH trial revealed significant improvement in one-year survival from 25% to 52%.with improvement of the quality of life in patients supported with VAD in comparison with optical medical therapy. In the post rematch era despite improvements in design, there was no significant improvement in clinical outcomes with pulsatile flow devices. Recently published Heart Mate II trial showed that patients supported with continuous flow HM II LVAD had significantly improved two-year survival when compared to pulsatile flow HM XVE recipients (58% vs. 24%, respectively) and significantly improved probability of freedom from stroke and device failure at two years, as compared to the recipients of pulsatile devices.

Experiences of the post-REMATCH era have shown that many DT recipients who were initially deemed not transplantable have improved their condition and became eligible for HT; 1 in every 5 recipients of HM XVE in the post-REMATCH era (17% of the 280 studied patients) underwent successful HT within 10 months from device implant. In most of these cases the improvements occurred due to the resolution of deemed irreversible pulmonary hypertension, recovery of renal function, weight loss, achieving cancer-free period, or reversal of other conditions. Therefore, one should not assume that DT would in the future preclude transplantation. Although LVAD implantation in the post-REMATCH era continues to be associated with substantial survival benefit as compared to medical therapy the outcomes of DT remain substantially inferior to those of HT (85% one-year survival).

6. Risk stratification and patient selection

Data from the REMATCH study[4] and the more recent post-REMATCH Registry,[8] of 300 recipients of the pulsatile HeartMate XVE device implanted as destination therapy since the close of REMATCH, as well as the HeartMate II trial[22] with the continuous flow pump in patients awaiting heart transplant, have all demonstrated that nearly 70% of the deaths in the first year occurred prior to hospital discharge. This finding is clearly independent of the pump design or indication for its use and reflects the very high severity of illness of these patients at the time of device implantation.[23]

The risk factors associated with death prior to hospital discharge were analyzed using data from the post-REMATCH Registry of destination therapy patients.[24] Those identified by multivariate analysis included platelets <149,000, prolonged coagulation (INR > 1.2), low pulmonary artery pressure (reflective of right ventricular failure), and importantly, malnutrition as evidenced by the crude marker of serum albumin <3.3 mg/dl. Hazard ratio was calculated for each of these preoperative laboratory variables, converted that hazard to a numerical score for each variable, and sum of these scores into a total risk score for in-hospital mortality was calculated. The data showed a tight linear correlation between higher risk score and increased in-hospital mortality, with high sensitivity and specificity. When the lowest-risk and medium risk cohorts were combined, the average survival was 70% at one year. For those with the highest risk score, the in-hospital mortality was >80% and a one-year survival was only 6%.

Many risk factors may be mitigated by intensive medical therapy; nutrition, coagulation profiles, right ventricular function, and renal function can be improved. Risk scoring can be used to select the optimal timing for device implantation. A patient with a very high or prohibitive risk score might undergo intensive medical management for a week, resulting in significant improvement in the risk score and a better outcome. These findings are based on the first generation of pulsatile pumps for destination therapy, but similar predictive accuracy has been recently reported in a large cohort of bridge-to-transplantation patients supported with both pulsatile and continuous-flow pumps.[24] If validated, the use of preoperative risk scoring will likely lead to improved outcomes with VADs.

7. Complications

Some of the most common perioperative complications of VAD placement include hemorrhage, right ventricular failure, sepsis, air embolism, and kinking of conduits. The late complications are mechanical device failure, neurologic events, and infection.[4,44,45]

7.1 Mechanical failure

Mechanical failure of VADs is an important cause of morbidity and mortality in patients living with VADs, because of the prolonged support required for both bridge to transplantation and destination therapy. The REMATCH trial has shown that 35% of patients experienced component failure within 24 months of implantation.[4] Another study on 109 patients with pulsatile VADs found that the probability of device failure was 6%, 12%, 27%, and 64% at 6 months, 1 year, 18 months, and 2 years, respectively.[46] On the other hand for continuous flow pumps the mechanical durability seems to be markedly improved. In one study on patients with a HeartMate II VAD as bridge to transplantation, only 5 of 133 (4%) developed either device thrombosis or a complication from surgical implantation necessitating device replacement.

Complications can arise in any component from the portable drive/system controller that controls and powers the device to the inflow and outflow cannulae, valves, batteries, and the VAD itself. These devices have system controllers and monitors that provide visual and auditory alarms during malfunction. To diagnose suspected device malfunction these alarms must be used in conjunction with clinical, laboratory, and imaging data. For troubleshooting, systematic catheter-, angiography-, fluoroscopy-, and echocardiography-based protocols have been developed to help diagnose common malfunctions.[47-50] If necessary, repair of a dysfunctional VAD or removal and replacement with a new VAD may be performed.

7.2 Neurologic events

Implanted mechanical devices are susceptible to thrombo-embolic events due to their unique properties. The foreign surfaces of VADs can activate the immune system, platelets, and the coagulation cascade. In addition, the blood-contact surfaces of VADs along with turbulent blood flow increase the risk of shear stress on blood and thrombi formation.[51] The unmasking or inadequate treatment of hypertension, older age, higher VAD flow and index, and inadequate anticoagulation further increase the risk for development of neurological events. Neurologic complications from VAD therapy include cerebro-vascular accidents and transient ischemic attacks, with an incidence ranging from 0.009 to 5.73 events per patient-year.[51,52] The prevalence of neurologic events with destination therapy has ranged from 44% in the REMATCH trial (HeartMate XVE) to 57% in the European LionHeart Clinical Utility Baseline Study. Intracranial hemorrhage, syncope, seizure, brain abscesses, and encephalopathy have all been reported. These data are mostly from the bridge-to-transplantation experience and may not apply to destination therapy patients who are generally older and have more co-morbidities and longer implantation periods.[53]

Not all devices have the same neurologic event rate. Design modifications like the use of novel biologic materials, textured coatings, and a single moving part, are believed to reduce the risk of thrombus formation. Promising data from the HeartMate II trial demonstrated reduced adverse events per patient year with respect to stroke (0.19 vs. 0.44) and non-stroke (0.26 vs. 0.67) neurologic events compared with a pulsatile flow pump[8]. Appropriate device selection, prevention of infection that can activate platelets, blood pressure control, and meticulous regulation of anticoagulation are all critical for the prevention of cerebro-vascular accidents after VAD implantation.[54,55]

7.3 Infection

VAD infections occur most frequently between 2 weeks and 2 months after implantation[56]. The predominant organisms are Gram-positive organisms *Staphylococcus epidermidis* and

Staphylococcus aureus followed by enterococci.[57-59] Other commonly implicated organisms include Gram negative bacilli such as *Pseudomonas aeruginosa, Enterobacter,* and *Klebsiella* species, along with fungi.[58,60] Frequent use of broad-spectrum antibiotics, particularly during the index hospitalization, is believed to increase susceptibility for fungal infections, which are associated with the highest risk of death.[60,61]

The most common site of infection is the percutaneous driveline, which can often be managed successfully with wound care and antibiotics.[62] However, a driveline infection can spread to other components of the VAD resulting in bacteremia, sepsis, and endocarditis[63]. Sepsis in patients with mechanical assist devices has been reported to be the leading cause of death and can result in cerebral emboli and multi-organ failure.[58,60] Other infections, including mediastinitis and peritonitis, have also been reported.

Many strategies have been adopted to try to minimize device-related and wound infections. Proper care of the driveline exit site must be maintained. Strict aseptic technique (e.g., sterile gloves, mask) must be followed when caring for the percutaneous exit site. The site should be gently cleaned with a mild antimicrobial soap and rinsed with sterile normal saline after which a dry sterile dressing should be applied. At all times, the driveline must be secured to minimize the risk of trauma; immobilization can be performed with an abdominal binder, additional gauze, tape, or a stoma-adhesive device.[64,65] There are also many modifications made to device design to further decrease the risk of infection which include the use of larger single-lead drivelines and drivelines coated with chlorhexidine and silver sulfadiazine.[60,66] Studies of rotary blood pumps with their reduced surface area for colonization and smaller surgical pump pocket suggest that they are less prone to infection.[67,68]

8. Future directions

The combination of VADs with adjunctive therapies may result in further improvement in ventricular function and lead to higher rates of clinical recovery. VADs provides an ideal platform to apply adjunctive therapies that directly target the causes of disease and potentially lead to myocardial regeneration and full restoration of function.[69] An adjunctive therapy that is best evaluated in patients with mechanical circulatory support is stem cell therapy. The clinical trials of cell therapy performed so far using autologous adult progenitor cells in acute myocardial infarction patients[70] have shown limited efficacy, with little information on the mechanisms responsible for the small functional improvement observed.[71] There is only less than 2% survival of transplanted cells in animals models present after two weeks post-transplant, and true cardiomyogenesis does not seem to occur.[72] From this it appears that paracrine mechanisms are most likely to account for the improvements in functional recovery of the recipient myocardium.[73] Other cell types, such as embryonic stem cells, inducible pluripotent stem cells, and cardiac progenitor cells, have larger potential for cardiac regeneration but their integration in the recipient myocardium remains a crucial problem.[74] Cell delivery is usually given either by intracoronary or by peripheral intravenous injection, with only a few patients undergoing direct delivery into the wall of the cardiac ventricle.[75] Having the heart directly exposed at the time of the VAD implant as a bridge-to-transplantation allows the direct intracardiac injection of a large number of cells into very specific mapped areas of the ventricle and provides an opportunity to study the direct effects at the histological and molecular levels when the heart is explanted for recovery or at time of transplant. In addition, the more favorable milieu offered by the VAD induced reverse remodeling, together with the reduced ventricular pressures, may promote the survival and integration of the injected cells, which would otherwise succumb in the hostile environment of the failing myocardium.

Gene therapy is also tried as an adjunctive therapy with VAD insertion, to manipulate critical genes differentially regulated in advanced heart failure[76,77]. Gene transfer can be achieved either by using viral vectors or by transfection into the patient's progenitor/ stem cells to be used for cell therapy, prior to VAD surgery. Gene therapy could directly target mechanisms responsible for heart failure, aim to enhance angiogenesis or myogenesis and protect the transplanted cells from apoptosis, and prevent the unloading-induced negative remodeling.

9. Conclusion

Though cardiac transplantation remains the gold standard for cardiac replacement therapy, as donor hearts are a very limited resource, alternatives in the form of mechanical assist devices have become a useful solution in treating patients with end stage heart failure. The field of VAD therapy is clearly expanding, being used as bridge to transplantation and as destination therapy. The new generation of continuous-flow pumps has yielded encouraging preliminary data suggesting both improved outcomes and device durability. The development of validated risk stratification models will lead to improved patient selection and timing of device implant, with overall improved outcomes over time. The novel adjunctive therapies like the stem cell transplant and the gene therapy may well usher in a new era of enhanced utilization of these devices for truly sustainable ventricular recovery as an alternative to life-long support.

10. References

[1] Lloyd-Jones D, Adams R, Carnethon M, et al. Heart disease and stroke statistics, 2009 update. A report from the american heart association statistics committee and stroke statistics subcommittee. *Circulation* 2009;119:e21-181.

[2] Miller LW, Missov ED. Epidemiology of heart failure. *Cardiol Clin* 2001;19:547-55.

[3] Park SJ, Tector A, Piccioni W, et al. Left ventricular assist devices as destination therapy: a new look at survival. *J Thorac Cardiovasc Surg* 2005;129:9-17.

[4] Rose EA, Gelijns AC, Moskowitz AJ, et al. Long-term mechanical left ventricular assistance for end-stage heart failure. *N Engl J Med* 2001;345:1435-43.

[5] Hershberger RE, Nauman D, Walker TL, et al. Care processes and clinical outcomes of continuous outpatient support with inotropes (COSI) in patients with refractory end stage heart failure. *J Card Fail* 2003;9:180-7.

[6] Fang J, Mensah GA, Croft JB, et al. Heart failure-related hospitalization in the U.S., 1979-2004. *J Am Coll Cardiol* 2008;52:428-34.

[7] Nose Y. Implantable total artificial heart developed by Abiomed gets FDA approval for clinical trials. *Artif Organs* 2001;25:429.

[8] Lietz K, Long JW, Kfoury AG, et al. Outcomes of left ventricular assist device implantation as destination therapy in the post-REMATCH era: implications for patient selection. *Circulation* 2007;116:497-505.

[9] Pagani FD, Miller LW, Russell SD, et al. 2009. Extended mechanical circulatory support with a continuous-flow rotary left ventricular assist device. *J. Am. Coll. Cardiol.* 54:312-21

[10] Christiansen S, Klocke A, Autschbach R. 2008. Past, present, and future of long-term mechanical cardiac support in adults. *J. Card. Surg.* 23:664–76

[11] Frazier OH, Benedict CR, Radovancevic B, et al. 1996. Improved left ventricular function after chronic left ventricular unloading. *Ann. Thorac. Surg.* 62:675–81

[12] Aharon AS, Drinkwater DC Jr, Churchwell KB, et al. 2001. Extracorporeal membrane oxygenation in children after repair of congenital cardiac lesions. *Ann. Thorac. Surg.* 72:2095–101

[13] Henriques JP, Remmelink M, Baan J Jr, et al. 2006. Safety and feasibility of elective high-risk percutaneous coronary intervention procedures with left ventricular support of the Impella Recover LP 2.5. *Am. J. Cardiol.* 97:990–92

[14] Thiele H, Lauer B, Hambrecht R, et al. 2001. Reversal of cardiogenic shock by percutaneous left atrialto- femoral arterial bypass assistance. *Circulation* 104:2917–22

[15] Henriques JP, de Mol BA. 2008. New percutaneous mechanical left ventricular support for acute MI: the AMC MACH program. *Nat. Clin. Pract. Cardiovasc. Med.* 5:62–63

[16] Mather PJ, Konstam MA. 2007. Newer mechanical devices in the management of acute heart failure. *Heart Fail. Rev.* 12:167–72

[17] Frazier OH, Rose EA, Oz MC, Dembitsky W, et al. Multicenter clinical evaluation of the HeartMate vented electric left ventricular assist system in patients awaiting heart transplantation. *J Thoracic Cardiovasc Surg* 2001; 122:1186–1195.

[18] Kalya AV, Tector AJ, Crouch JD, et al. Comparison of Novacor and HeartMate vented electric left ventricular assist devices in single institution. *J Heart Lung Transplant* 2005; 24:1973–1975.

[19] El-Banayosy A, Arusoglu L, Kizner L, et al. Novacor left ventricular assist systems versus HeartMate vented electric left ventricular system as a long mechanical support device in bridging patients: a prospective study. *J Thoracic Cardiovasc Surg* 2000; 119:581–587.

[20] Esmore D, Kaye D, Spratt P, et al. A prospective, multicenter trial of the VentrAssist left ventricular assist device for bridge to transplant, safety and efficacy. *J Heart Lung Transplant* 2008; 27:579–588.

[21] Morshuis M, El-Banayosy A, Arusoglu L, et al. European experience of DuraHeart magnetically levitated centrifugal left ventricular assist system. *Eur J Cardiothorac Surg* 2009; 35:1020–1028

[22] Miller LW, Pagani FD, Russell SD, et al. 2007. Use of a continuous-flow device in patients awaiting heart transplantation. *N. Engl. J. Med.* 357:885–96

[23] Miller LW, Lietz K. 2006. Candidate selection for long-term left ventricular assist device therapy forrefractory heart failure. *J. Heart Lung Transplant.* 25:756–64

[24] Lietz K, Long JW, Kfoury AG, et al. 2007. Outcomes of left ventricular assist device implantation as destination therapy in the post-REMATCH era: implications for patient selection. *Circulation* 116:497–505

[25] Kaye DM, Hoshijima M, Chien KR. 2008. Reversing advanced heart failure by targeting Ca_2^+ cycling. *Annu. Rev. Med.* 59:13–28

[26] Terracciano CM, Harding SE, Adamson D, et al. 2003. Changes in sarcolemmal Ca entry and sarcoplasmic reticulum Ca content in ventricular myocytes from patients with end-stage heart failure following myocardial recovery after combined pharmacological and ventricular assist device therapy. *Eur. Heart J.* 24:1329-39

[27] Dipla K, Mattiello JA, Jeevanandam V, et al. 1998. Myocyte recovery after mechanical circulatory support in humans with end-stage heart failure. *Circulation* 97:2316–22

[28] Heerdt PM, Holmes JW, Cai B, et al. 2000. Chronic unloading by left ventricular assist device reverses contractile dysfunction and alters gene expression in end-stage heart failure. *Circulation* 102:2713–19

[29] Ogletree-Hughes ML, Stull LB, Sweet WE, et al. 2001. Mechanical unloading restores beta-adrenergic responsiveness and reverses receptor downregulation in the failing human heart. *Circulation* 104:881–86

[30] Terracciano CM, Hardy J, Birks EJ, et al. 2004. Clinical recovery from end-stage heart failure using leftventricular assist device and pharmacological therapy correlates with increased sarcoplasmic reticulum calcium content but not with regression of cellular hypertrophy. *Circulation* 109:2263–65

[31] Harding JD, Piacentino V III, Gaughan JP, et al. 2001. Electrophysiological alterations after mechanical circulatory support in patients with advanced cardiac failure. *Circulation* 104:1241–47

[32] Xydas S, Rosen RS, Ng C, et al. 2006. Mechanical unloading leads to echocardiographic, electrocardiographic, neurohormonal, and histologic recovery. *J. Heart Lung Transplant.* 25:7–15

[33] Maybaum S, Mancini D, Xydas S, et al. 2007. Cardiac improvement during mechanical circulatory support: a prospective multicenter study of the LVADWorking Group. *Circulation* 115:2497–505

[34] Mancini DM, Beniaminovitz A, Levin H, et al. 1998. Low incidence of myocardial recovery after left ventricular assist device implantation in patients with chronic heart failure. *Circulation* 98:2383–89

[35] Ritter M, Su Z, Xu S, et al. 2000. Cardiac unloading alters contractility and calcium homeostasis in ventricular myocytes. *J. Mol. Cell Cardiol.* 32:577–84

[36] Kolar F, MacNaughton C, Papousek F, et al. 1995. Changes in calcium handling in atrophic heterotopically isotransplanted rat hearts. *Basic Res. Cardiol.* 90:475–81

[37] Welsh DC, Dipla K, McNulty PH, et al. 2001. Preserved contractile function despite atrophic remodelling in unloaded rat hearts. *Am. J. Physiol. Heart Circ. Physiol.* 281:H1131-36

[38] Oriyanhan W, Tsuneyoshi H, Nishina T, et al. 2007. Determination of optimal duration of mechanical unloading for failing hearts to achieve bridge to recovery in a rat heterotopic heart transplantation model. *J. Heart Lung Transplant.* 26:16–23

[39] Ito K, Nakayama M, Hasan F, et al. 2003. Contractile reserve and calcium regulation are depressed in myocytes from chronically unloaded hearts. *Circulation* 107:1176–82

[40] Soppa GK, Lee J, Stagg MA, et al. 2008. Prolonged mechanical unloading reduces myofilament sensitivity to calcium and sarcoplasmic reticulum calcium uptake leading to contractile dysfunction. *J. Heart Lung Transplant.* 27:882–89

[41] Yacoub MH. 2001. A novel strategy to maximize the efficacy of left ventricular assist devices as a bridge to recovery. *Eur. Heart J.* 22:534–40

[42] Soppa GK, SmolenskiRT, Latif N, et al. 2005. Effects of chronic administration of clenbuterol on function and metabolism of adult rat cardiac muscle. *Am. J. Physiol. Heart Circ. Physiol.* 288:H1468–76

[43] Birks EJ, Tansley PD, Hardy J, et al. 2006. Left ventricular assist device and drug therapy for the reversal of heart failure. *N. Engl. J. Med.* 355:1873–84

[44] Gordon RJ, Quagliarello B, Lowy FD. Ventricular assist devicerelated infections. *Lancet Infect Dis* 2006;6:426 –37.

[45] Piccione W Jr. Left ventricular assist device implantation: short and long-term surgical complications. *J Heart Lung Transplant* 2000;19: S89–94.

[46] Birks EJ, Tansley PD, Yacoub MH, et al. Incidence and clinical management of life-threatening left ventricular assist device failure. *J Heart Lung Transplant* 2004;23:964 –9.

[47] Horton SC, Khodaverdian R, Chatelain P, et al. Left ventricular assist device malfunction: an approach to diagnosis by echocardiography. *J Am Coll Cardiol* 2005;45:1435– 40.

[48] Catena E, Milazzo F, Montorsi E, et al. Left ventricular support by axial flow pump: the echocardiographic approach to device malfunction. *J Am Soc Echocardiogr* 2005;18:1422, e7–13.

[49] Horton SC, Khodaverdian R, Powers A, et al. Left ventricular assist device malfunction: a systematic approach to diagnosis. *J Am Coll Cardiol* 2004;43:1574–83.

[50] Scalia GM, McCarthy PM, Savage RM, Smedira NG, Thomas JD. Clinical utility of echocardiography in the management of implantable ventricular assist devices. *J Am Soc Echocardiogr* 2000;13:754–63.

[51] Pae WE, Connell JM, Boehmer JP, et al. Neurologic events with a totally implantable left ventricular assist device: European LionHeart Clinical Utility Baseline Study (CUBS). *J Heart Lung Transplant* 2007;26:1– 8.

[52] Thomas CE, Jichici D, Petrucci R, Urrutia VC, Schwartzman RJ. Neurologic complications of the Novacor left ventricular assist device. *Ann Thorac Surg* 2001;72:1311–5.

[53] Lazar RM, Shapiro PA, Jaski BE, et al. Neurological events during long-term mechanical circulatory support for heart failure: the Randomized Evaluation of Mechanical Assistance for the Treatment of Congestive Heart Failure (REMATCH) experience. *Circulation* 2004;109:2423–7.

[54] Tsukui H, Abla A, Teuteberg JJ, et al. Cerebrovascular accidents in patients with a ventricular assist device. *J Thorac Cardiovasc Surg* 2007;134:114 –23.

[55] Slaughter MS, Sobieski MA, Gallagher C, Dia M, Silver MA. Low incidence of neurologic events during long-term support with the HeartMate XVE left ventricular assist device. *Tex Heart Inst J* 2008;35:245–9.

[56] Simon D, Fischer S, Grossman A, et al. Left ventricular assist device-related infection: treatment and outcome. *Clin Infect Dis* 2005;40:1108 –15.

[57] Kalya AV, Tector AJ, Crouch JD, et al. Comparison of Novacor and HeartMate vented electric left ventricular assist devices in a single institution. *J Heart Lung Transplant* 2005;24:1973–5.

[58] Sivaratnam K, Duggan JM. Left ventricular assist device infections: three case reports and a review of the literature. *Asaio J* 2002;48:2-7.

[59] Sinha P, Chen JM, Flannery M, Scully BE, Oz MC, Edwards NM. Infections during left ventricular assist device support do not affect posttransplant outcomes. Circulation 2000;102:III194 -9.

[60] Gordon SM, Schmitt SK, Jacobs M, et al. Nosocomial bloodstreaminfections in patients with implantable left ventricular assist devices. *Ann Thorac Surg* 2001;72:725–30.

[61] Nurozler F, Argenziano M, Oz MC, Naka Y. Fungal left ventricular assist device endocarditis. *Ann Thorac Surg* 2001;71:614–8.

[62] Robbins RC, Kown MH, Portner PM, Oyer PE. The totally implantable Novacor left ventricular assist system. *Ann Thorac Surg* 2001;71: S162–5.

[63] Holman WL, Park SJ, Long JW, et al. Infection in permanent circulatory support: experience from the REMATCH trial. *J Heart Lung Transplant* 2004;23:1359–65.

[64] Chinn R, Dembitsky W, Eaton L, et al. Multicenter experience: prevention and management of left ventricular assist device infections. *Asaio J* 2005;51:461–70.

[65] Pasque MK, Hanselman T, Shelton K, et al. Surgical management of Novacor drive-line exit site infections. *Ann Thorac Surg* 2002;74: 1267–8.

[66] Zierer A, Melby SJ, Voeller RK, et al. Late-onset driveline infections: the Achilles' heel of prolonged left ventricular assist device support. *Ann Thorac Surg* 2007;84:515–20.

[67] Siegenthaler MP, Martin J, Pernice K, et al. The Jarvik 2000 is associated with less infections than the HeartMate left ventricular assist device. *Eur J Cardiothorac Surg* 2003;23:748 -54.

[68] Vitali E, Lanfranconi M, Ribera E, et al. Successful experience in bridging patients to heart transplantation with the MicroMed De- Bakey ventricular assist device. *Ann Thorac Surg* 2003;75:1200–4.

[69] Renlund DG, Kfoury AG. 2006. When the failing, end-stage heart is not end-stage. *N. Engl. J. Med.* 355:1922–25

[70] Abdel-Latif A, Bolli R, Tleyjeh IM, et al. 2007. Adult bone marrow-derived cells for cardiac repair: a systematic review and meta-analysis. *Arch. Intern. Med.* 167:989–97

[71] Dimmeler S, Zeiher AM, Schneider MD. 2005. Unchain my heart: the scientific foundations of cardiac repair. *J. Clin. Invest.* 115:572–83

[72] Murry CE, Soonpaa MH, Reinecke H, et al. 2004. Haematopoietic stem cells do not transdifferentiate into cardiac myocytes in myocardial infarcts. *Nature* 428:664–68

[73] Lee J, Stagg MA, Fukushima S, et al. 2009. Adult progenitor cell transplantation influences contractile performance and calcium handling of recipient cardiomyocytes. *Am. J. Physiol. Heart Circ. Physiol.* 296:H927–36

[74] van Laake LW, Passier R, Doevendans PA, et al. 2008. Human embryonic stem cell-derived cardiomyocytes and cardiac repair in rodents. *Circ. Res.* 102:1008–10

[75] Menasche P, Alfieri O, Janssens S, et al. 2008. The Myoblast Autologous Grafting in Ischemic Cardiomyopathy (MAGIC) trial: first randomized placebo-controlled study of myoblast transplantation. *Circulation* 117:1189–200

[76] Schneider MD, French BA. 1993. The advent of adenovirus. Gene therapy for cardiovascular disease. *Circulation* 88:1937–42

[77] Murtuza B, Suzuki K, Bou-Gharios G, et al. 2004. Transplantation of skeletal myoblasts secreting an IL-1 inhibitor modulates adverse remodeling in infarcted murine myocardium. *Proc. Natl. Acad. Sci. USA* 101:4216–21

[78] Barry A. Boilson, MB, MRCPI, MD, Eugenia Raichlin, MD, Soon J. Park, MD, and Sudhir S. Kushwaha, MD: Device Therapy and Cardiac Transplantation for End-Stage Heart Failure; *Curr Probl Cardiol*, January 2010

[79] Cesare M. Terracciano, LeslieW. Miller, and Magdi H. Yacoub: Contemporary Use of Ventricular Assist Devices. *Annu. Rev. Med* 2010

[80] Sean R. Wilson, MD, Michael M. Givertz, MD, Garrick C. Stewart, MD, Gilbert H. Mudge, JR, MD. Ventricular Assist DevicesThe Challenges of Outpatient Management; *Journal of American College of Cardiology* Vol 54, No 18, 2009.

[81] J.R. Lahpor: State of the art: implantable ventricular assist devices; *Current Opinion in Organ Transplantation* 2009, 14:554–559.

[82] Katherine Lietz, M.D., Ph.D. Destination Therapy: Patient Selection and Current Outcomes; *J Card Surg* 2010;25:462-471

5

Myocardial Recovery Following Left Ventricular Assist Device Therapy

M. Navaratnarajah, M. Ibrahim, M. Yacoub and C. Terracciano
Heart Science Centre, Imperial College London, Harefield Hospital
United Kingdom

1. Introduction

Heart Failure (HF) represents an increasing clinical problem with a reported mortality (for either diastolic or systolic HF) of approximately 60% at 5 years after diagnosis (Shahar et al. 2004). The incidence of end-stage HF has increased four-fold in the last 20 years (Hubler et al. 2003; Terracciano et al. 2010). Symptomatic HF confers a worse prognosis than the majority of cancers, with mortality as high as 45% at one year (Cohn 1996; Jessup and Brozena 2003), and there are currently more than 16 million people in Europe and the United States (US) suffering from this disease. HF is also a major burden in the developing world (Mayosi 2007). Despite substantial medical advances in the treatment of HF, cardiac transplantation (CTx) remains the best long term therapy for patients suffering from end-stage disease, with 50 % survival at 10 years post CTx (Hunt, SA et al. 2009a; Trulock et al. 2007). A fixed and inadequate donor organ pool means that CTx is available to only a small proportion of eligible patients. In the US an estimated 100 000 patients are believed to be suitable for CTx (Maybaum et al. 2008), but only 2200 transplants are performed annually (Hunt,SA et al. 2009b). As a consequence the use of LVADs as Bridge-to-Transplantation (BTT) has increased steadily over the last few years and approximately 9000 CTx candidates, i.e. more than a third of all listed candidates in the US, have undergone LVAD implantation since 1999 (Mancini and Lietz 2010).

Initially, LVADs were utilised in the acute setting, in the management of post-cardiotomy cardiogenic shock (PCCS), a rare clinical scenario associated with high morbidity and mortality (Mehta et al. 1996). Despite improvements in LVAD technology, and the understanding of PCCS, the use of mechanical unloading (MU) in this acute setting is now minimal, with large studies showing survival of 23-52.4% (Sylvin et al. 2010).

The role of LVADs subsequently expanded to incorporate patients with severe drug-resistant HF, primarily as a BTT, with subsequent extension of the role to include "destination therapy" (DT) in those patients unsuitable for CTx (Kirklin et al. 2011).

In a small minority of patients a third application for chronic LVAD therapy, "Bridge-to-Recovery" (BTR) evolved, following the observation that MU appeared to coincide with cellular, molecular, electrophysiological and structural myocardial changes consistent with functional recovery (Altemose et al. 1997; Farrar et al. 2002; Heerdt,PM et al. 2000a; Hetzer et al. 2000; Ogletree-Hughes et al. 2001; Sylvin et al. 2010; Young 2001). Such observations allied with anecdotal examples of cardiac recovery in isolated patients following enforced device removal (mandated by the development of complications) (Frazier 1994; Frazier and

Myers 1999), alerted the world to the possibility that the remodelling of end-stage HF was reversible ("reverse remodelling") (Klotz et al. 2008).
Within the context of an increasing incidence of HF, amongst a growing population of older patients (> 65 yrs) ineligible to receive CTx, inadequate organ availability and ever improving pump technology, the concept of BTR offers great hope as a potential treatment strategy to either replace, or work alongside that of CTx in years to come. However, BTR i.e. sufficient recovery of cardiac function to allow explantation of device, remains a controversial subject, with few successful reported cases worldwide(Birks et al. 2006; Birks et al. 2011; Maybaum et al. 2007). The Harefield protocol, a novel strategy in which LVAD is combined with pharmacotherapy including the β_2-AR agonist Clenbuterol, significantly increases the rate of explantation (Birks *et al.*, 2006;Birks *et al.*, 2011; see section 6 of this Chapter). In general, explantation rates vary considerably between studies but, with the exception of the Harefield protocol, remain universally low within the context of chronic HF (Dandel et al. 2005; Simon et al. 2005).
The purpose of this chapter is to review the effects of LVAD therapy, focussing on the mechanisms mediating functional recovery. We review clinical and experimental data supporting and opposing the concept of BTR. The first section of this chapter will focus on myocardial reverse remodelling followed by the clinical aspects of BTR.

2. Myocardial reverse remodelling

Myocardial remodelling associated with LVAD therapy is known to occur at structural, whole heart, cellular, molecular, metabolic, electrophysiological, cell survival and functional levels.

2.1 LVAD induced reverse structural remodelling

2.1.1 Restoration of cardiac geometry and regression of myocyte hypertrophy

LVAD therapy has been shown to reduce left ventricular dimensions (Frazier et al. 1996) and to restore the end-diastolic-pressure volume relationships (EDPVR) towards normal values (Levin et al. 1995). In addition, regression of both cardiac and myocyte hypertrophy has been consistently demonstrated to occur during LVAD treatment (Madigan et al. 2001; Zafeiridis et al. 1998).
Pharmacotherapy alone has proved effective in retarding the negative remodelling associated with HF (Yancy et al. 2001), but is unable to induce profound reverse remodelling to the extent of LVAD therapy (Levin et al. 1995). The structural changes described have not been documented in the right ventricle (RV) of LVAD supported patients, suggesting that the predominant factor driving remodelling to be haemodynamic (Klotz et al. 2008), rather than the normalization of neurohumoral and cytokine environment known to occur during support (Birks et al. 2001; Delgado, III et al. 1998; Klotz et al. 2009; McCarthy et al. 1995).

2.1.2 Cytoskeletal proteins

Sarcomeric and skeletal protein changes have been consistently shown to occur in association with MU. De Jonge *et al.* demonstrated improvements in distorted cytoskeletal architecture involving a number of proteins including actin, tropomyosin, troponin T and troponin C (De et al. 2002). Reversal of disruption of the amino terminus of dystrophin (Vatta et al. 2004), and upregulation of dystrophin gene expression (Mohapatra et al. 2010) occur in LVAD supported patients. Work conducted at Harefield hospital demonstrated a specific collection of protein expression alterations that coincided with functional recovery and device explantation, involving a variety of proteins such as myosin heavy chain, sarcomeric actin, troponin C, troponin T, lamin A/C , spectrin, integrins beta1, beta6, alpha-tropomyosin, alpha1-actinin, and vinculin (Birks et al. 2005; Latif et al. 2007).

2.1.3 Extracellular matrix

The ECM constitutes approximately 3 % of normal myocardium, and is largely made up of collagen. Type 1 collagen, type 1: type 3 collagen ratio, collagen cross linking and fibrosis have been shown to be elevated in a variety of clinical as well as experimental disease states (Avendano et al. 1999; Badenhorst et al. 2003; Marijianowski et al. 1995; Mukherjee and Sen 1991; Porter and Turner 2009; Woodiwiss et al. 2001).

Reports of LVAD-induced ECM changes have been conflicting, with some revealing increased myocardial fibrosis and ECM volume following unloading (Klotz, S. et al. 2005b; Li et al. 2001; Matsumiya et al. 2005; Saito et al. 2010), and others showing a reduction (Akgul et al. 2004; Bruckner et al. 2001; Maybaum et al. 2007; Thohan et al. 2005; Thompson et al. 2005). Bruggink *et al.* demonstrated a biphasic response with initial expansion of ECM and then a subsequent regression with prolonged MU (Bruggink et al. 2006). This discrepancy is thought to arise from differences in HF aetiology, duration of MU, pharmacotherapy employed during MU (Klotz,S et al. 2007a), as well as the varying and often semi-quantitative methods utilised for analysis (Bruckner et al. 2000).

Matrix metalloproteinases (MMPs) are a group of enzymes responsible for collagen degradation and are tightly regulated by tissue inhibitors of metalloproteinases (TIMPs). HF is associated with large changes in MMP and TIMP action and thus ECM composition (Li et al. 2001; Matsumiya et al. 2005), and it is understood that altered regulation in their expression contributes to "negative" ECM remodelling in HF (Mann and Spinale 1998; Spinale et al. 2000; Wilson and Spinale 2001). Normalisation (decrease) of MMP1:TIMP1 ratio has been reported with LVAD use in a DCM population and coincides with increased LV collagen cross linking, type 1: type 3 ratio and increased ventricular stiffness (Klotz,S et al. 2005b). A study conducted at Harefield hospital showed that all but one (TIMP4) of the MMPs and TIMPs studied, displayed a change in expression during LVAD therapy (Felkin et al. 2009). TIMP4 expression decreased in this study in contrast to previous studies showing unchanged/decreased MMP and augmented TIMP levels to coincide with LVAD support (Klotz,S et al. 2005b; Li et al. 2001). Levels of cardiac fibrosis (Matsumiya et al. 2005; Saito et al. 2010) and profibrotic marker gene expression (Felkin et al. 2009) at time of LVAD implantation demonstrate predictive power with regards to likelihood of subsequent functional recovery, device explantability and durability of recovery. Negative ECM remodelling may represent a potentially important modifiable barrier to recovery in HF patients (Klotz, S. et al., 2007b).

Pharmacological blockade of the Renin-Angiotensin-Aldosterone-System (RAAS) in HF therapy is known to decrease cardiac fibrosis, collagen content and ventricular dilatation, with significant improvements in mortality (Arnold et al. 2003). Similar effects on ECM have also been seen in several different experimental models of HF (Bartha et al. 2008; Ibrahim et al. 2009; Meng et al. 2009). Klotz et al. have shown that ACE inhibition (ACE-I) reduces the increase in LV myocardial Angiotensin II/noradrenaline (NA) (Klotz et al. 2009), total collagen levels and collagen crosslinking associated with LVAD therapy, leading to their suggestion that pharmacological manipulation of the ECM represents a critical target in improving the frequency and extent of recovery during LVAD therapy (Klotz, S. et al. 2007b).

No changes in RV chamber size, mass or collagen content were noted despite normalisation of MMP:TIMP ratio and myocardial Ang II levels, inferring that neither haemodynamic unloading nor pharmacotherapy alone were sufficient for positive structural ECM remodelling to occur, and that complex dual regulation (neurohumoral and haemodynamic) of fibrotic mechanisms is likely to exist. All patients were bridged to CTx in this retrospective study and hence the impact of these structural ECM changes on whole heart cardiac functional recovery was not assessed.

2.2 LVAD effects on Ca^{2+} regulation and signaling pathways

2.2.1 Ca^{2+} regulation

HF is associated with alterations in a multitude of Ca^{2+} regulatory mechanisms, the balance of which varies with stage and aetiology of disease (Bers 2006). Mishandling of cytoplasmic Ca^{2+} causes deranged myocyte excitation-contraction (EC) coupling, abnormal systolic and diastolic function, as well as arrythmogenesis in clinical and experimental HF (Gwathmey et al. 1987; Pieske et al. 1996). LVAD therapy is associated with reversal or alteration in expression and function, of many Ca^{2+} handling elements known to be adversely remodelled during HF, with a clear correlation with functional recovery being observed with certain parameters. Despite this, the true functional relevance of many of the LVAD- associated changes in Ca^{2+}cycling remains unclear.

Reverse electrophysiological remodelling occurs during LVAD therapy, demonstrated by reduction of QT interval and myocyte action potential duration (APD) (Harding et al. 2001). Mechanisms regulating APD involve alteration in function and expression of ion transporters with changes in depolarising and hyperpolarising currents. Detrimental effects of APD prolongation in HF on EC coupling, cellular relaxation and contraction are recognized (Gaughan et al. 1999; Wickenden et al. 1998), as well as positive effects such as augmentation of intracellular Ca^{2+} via alteration in L-type Ca^{2+} and NCX currents, presumed to be compensatory adaptive mechanisms (Bouchard et al. 1995; Weber et al. 2002; Wickenden et al. 1998). APD reduction has been associated with functional clinical recovery during LVAD support (Terracciano et al. 2004), but delineation of a precise contributory role of APD to functional recovery is difficult as the specific role of APD changes in HF itself remains unclear.

2.2.2 Sarcoplasmic reticulum Ca^{2+} content

A key determinant of effective Ca^{2+} release and myocyte contractility is the sarcoplasmic reticulum (SR) Ca^{2+} content and this parameter has been shown to be decreased in HF (Bers 2006) although increased SR Ca^{2+} content is noted to occur in some models during compensated HF (Soppa et al. 2008). 3 main mechanisms are thought to be responsible for the diminished SR Ca^{2+} content in HF : a) depressed Serca 2a function b) enhanced NCX function and c) enhanced SR Ca^{2+} leak (Bers 2006). Increased SR Ca^{2+} uptake has been shown to occur in response to LVAD support (Dipla et al. 1998; Frazier et al. 1996), and together with augmented Ca^{2+} transient amplitude correlate with improved myocyte contractility (Chaudhary et al. 2004; Dipla et al. 1998). Importantly, recovery of diminished SR Ca^{2+} content and L-type fast inactivation (most likely secondary to increased SR Ca^{2+} release) correlated with myocardial recovery and device explantation (Terracciano et al. 2004).

2.2.3 Serca 2a

Sarcoplasmic Endoreticulum Ca^{2+} ATPase 2a (SERCA 2a) is the principal protein responsible for the reuptake of Ca^{2+} into the SR, which allows for sufficient replenishing of Ca^{2+} stores for the subsequent heartbeat. Effects on Serca 2a gene expression and protein levels vary. Clinical and experimental studies have shown recovery (Takaseya et al. 2004), as well as no change (Chaudhary et al. 2004) to occur with MU, in addition to a biphasic response, i.e. initial recovery followed by subsequent decline coinciding with contractile function deterioration (Oriyanhan et al. 2007). Similarly, phospholamban (PLB) PLB:Serca2a ratio a key determinant of contractile function (Koss et al. 1997), known to be elevated in HF, displays a similar short term recovery (decreased ratio), with later resurgence of ratio coinciding with prolonged support and decline in contractile function (Ogletree et al. 2010).

2.2.4 Na^+-Ca^{2+} exchanger (NCX)

Enhanced NCX activity / gene expression and protein levels are known to occur in most but not all models of HF (Bers 2006) with certain studies showing no change(Hasenfuss et al. 1999; Komuro et al. 1992) or even a reduction (Heerdt,PM et al. 2000b). In an environment of high intracellular Na^+, prolonged APD and diminished Ca^{2+} transients, enhanced NCX activity promotes Ca^{2+} entry, a probable inotropic action. Reported LVAD-induced NCX changes are equivocal, improved Ca^{2+} extrusion has been associated with increased NCX gene expression and functional recovery (Terracciano et al. 2007). However, partial restoration of positive force frequency relationship (FFR) (Chaudhary et al. 2004), as well as enhanced contractile strength in non-recovered patients (Heerdt,PM et al. 2000a), occurs in the absence of alterations in NCX protein levels. The well documented discordance between gene expression and protein levels, as well as regional LV expression heterogeneity, may be responsible for such discrepancies.

2.2.5 Ryanodine receptor (RyR)

Diastolic Ca^{2+} leak secondary to deranged RyR function is also an important contributor in Ca^{2+} mishandling in HF(Marx et al. 2000). Chronic PKA mediated hyperphosphorylation of RyR2 promoting a "leaky" receptor is just one of the proposed mechanisms thought to lead to SR Ca^{2+} depletion and disease progression in HF (Kushnir and Marks 2010; Shan et al. 2010), and normalisation of this parameter has been seen to occur with LVAD support(Marx et al. 2000).

2.2.6 Beta-adrenergic signalling

Improvement of beta-AR (β-AR) responsiveness and density occurs during LVAD therapy (Dipla et al. 1998; Klotz, S. et al. 2005a; Milting et al. 2006; Ogletree-Hughes et al. 2001), as well as mechanically unloaded failing rat hearts (Oriyanhan et al. 2007). LVAD induced β-AR "recovery" is independent of cessation of systemic β-AR agonist therapy (Ogletree-Hughes et al. 2001), of greater magnitude than that caused by pharmacotherapy alone (Klotz, S. et al. 2005a), and unrelated to duration of support (Ogletree-Hughes et al. 2001). Mechanisms promoting such recovery remain unclear and direct haemodynamic unloading and/or normalisation of cytokine and neurohumoral environment are likely to be important. Support for the the latter as the predominant governing factor is derived from results showing LVAD associated β-AR recovery to occur in both RV and LV, despite isolated LV haemodynamic unloading (Klotz, S. et al. 2005b). Alteration in the specific expression of genes involved in β-AR signalling such as phosphodiesterase 1A, 3B, calcineurin A and Rap guanine nucleotide exchange factor 4 RAPGEF4 (EPAC2) has been shown to coincide with functional myocardial recovery in patients undergoing device explantation (Hall et al. 2007).

2.2.7 Neurohumoral effects

LVAD support is known to decrease plasma adrenaline, noradrenaline (NA), renin, aldosterone and vasopressin (Klotz et al. 2009) as well as Atrial and B-type natriuretic peptide plasma levels (Thompson et al. 2005), myocardial gene (Kuhn et al. 2004) and protein (Wohlschlaeger et al. 2008) expression. Occasional correlation between measured biomarkers and functional improvement raises the possibility of the potential use of such markers in guiding therapy and prediction of recovery (Thompson et al. 2005). However, LVAD effects on the RAAS have recently been shown to be complex, with actual increased myocardial Ang II and NA levels, occurring despite reductions in plasma renin and aldosterone levels (Klotz et al. 2009). Such changes are postulated to arise from an LVAD induced recovery of depleted angiotensinogen levels, leading to enhanced generation of myocardial Ang II with subsequent sympathetic stimulation causing elevated NA levels, and shown to correlate with increased fibrosis and ventricular stiffness (Klotz et al. 2009), structural changes that were prevented by ACE-I. The negative effects of NA and Ang II on ECM remodelling and apoptosis are well known (Bonnefont-Rousselot et al. 2002; Klotz, S. et al. 2007b), and such findings emphasise the importance of possible pharmacological manipulation of specific neuroendocrine pathways in combination with LVADs in promoting positive remodelling.

2.3 Cell survival and regeneration

2.3.1 Apoptosis

LVAD therapy appears to have beneficial effects on cell survival and apoptotic pathways although results are not uniform amongst studies. There are several distinct apoptotic pathways and their regulation is complex. Human HF is generally characterised by loss of cardiomyocytes (Narula et al. 2006) but rarely and inconsistently the presence of abundant apoptosis is demonstrated (Francis GS 1999).LVAD support causes normalisation and augmentation of anti-apoptotic proteins FasExo6Del (Bartling et al. 1999), BCL-XL levels (Milting et al. 1999), BCL-2 (Francis et al. 1999), decreased myocardial TNF-α levels (Razeghi et al. 2001; Torre-Amione et al. 1999), a cytokine believed to possess apoptotic regulatory properties , decreases in markers of DNA fragmentation (Bartling et al. 1999), cellular repair (PCNA) (Francis et al. 1999) and markers of cellular apoptosis(Baba et al. 2000).

2.3.2 Cardiomyocyte regeneration

LVAD-induced recovery of pro-apoptotic pathways activated in HF seemingly infers a potential for increased cell survival and augmentation of myocyte number, a mechanism that easily lends itself to promoting improved cardiac function and recovery. Previously held assumptions that cardiomyocytes are terminally differentiated, with severely limited, if any, potential to undergo mitotic division have now been challenged (Anversa and Kajstura 1998). Evidence showing that in response to injury cardiomyocyte division occurs (Beltrami et al. 2001; Engel et al. 2006), coupled to work demonstrating the existence of endogenous cardiac stem pools (Hosoda et al. 2010; Leri et al. 2005; Urbanek et al. 2005) naturally leads to the idea that together with the "anti-apoptotic" effects of LVAD therapy, the favourable biochemical and haemodynamic environment afforded by MU may also promote cardiac regeneration via increased cardiomyocyte division, or endogenous stem cell proliferation, thus reversing HF myocyte loss.

Evidence in support of such an LVAD role is limited (Wohlschlaeger et al. 2010). Wohlschlaeger et al. recently showed a dramatic 2 fold reduction in mean cardiomyocyte DNA and a 2 fold increase in number of diploid cardiomyocytes, together with significant decrease in the number of polyploid cardiomyocytes, a characteristic of human cardiac hypertrophy (Adler and Sandritter 1980; Sandritter and Adler 1976; Wohlschlaeger et al. 2010). The authors propose that these findings can be explained by a single unifying theory, hypothesising LVAD support to a) ameliorate hypertrophic stimuli that promote the transition of "mitotically arrested" cardiomyocytes into the S phase of DNA replication (Busk et al. 2002) (reduction in polyploidy), as well as b) promote real cell division or progenitor cell proliferation (increase in diploidy and reduction of DNA content per cardiomyocyte). Such findings require further mechanistic study, but clearly demonstrate the plasticity and reversibility of the cardiomyocyte DNA phenotype in HF, and raise the attractive possibility of LVAD-induced cardiac regeneration.

2.4 Myocardial metabolism and energetics

Myocardial metabolism and energetics have been shown to be consistently altered in HF (Neubauer 2007), resulting in an energy deficient mechanically inefficient heart, characterised by diminished ATP and phosphocreatine levels (Ingwall and Weiss 2004; Starling et al. 1998). The exact mechanisms remain unclear, but altered carbohydrate metabolism and myocardial insulin resistance have been proposed as key determinants of deranged energetics in HF and a potential therapeutic target (Ashrafian et al. 2007). LVAD therapy has been associated with improved mitochondrial metabolic function (Lee et al. 1998), and normalisation of mitochondrial cardiolipin constitution in ICM (Heerdt et al. 2002).. In addition, normalisation of raised myocardial Arginine:glycine amidinotransferase (AGAT) mRNA levels, occurs in patients successfully undergoing LVAD explantation as part of the Harefield protocol (Hall et al. 2007), reinforcing the importance of altered metabolic pathways in HF pathogenesis and future therapy.

2.5 IGF-1

Insulin growth factor (IGF-1) has been shown to possess favourable cardiac effects in experimental models of HF, with both early and delayed short term IGF-1 administration causing cardiac hypertrophy and improvement in function (Duerr et al. 1995; Duerr et al. 1996). IGF-1 displays anti-apoptotic (Li et al. 1997) as well as regenerative properties in both skeletal (Musaro 2005; Pelosi et al. 2007) and cardiac muscle (Santini et al. 2007; Welch et al. 2002), with cardiac specific IGF-1 expression attenuating disease progression in a mouse model of DCM (Welch et al. 2002).

IGF-1 mRNA levels are elevated at time of explantation of LVAD in patients treated with the Harefield protocol, suggesting elevated IGF-1 levels maybe important for the recovery process (Barton et al. 2005). 2 clearly defined groups were identified: those in which IGF-1 mRNA was high at implantation in which it remained high, and those in which IGF-1 mRNA was low at implantation and increased significantly during recovery. It is highly likely that the increase in IGF-1 mRNA seen in this study is induced by the combination therapy used in the Harefield protocol, and not MU alone, as previous studies have shown no change in IGF-1 expression or IGF pathway activation during isolated LVAD support in patients bridged to transplantation (Hall et al. 2004; Razeghi et al. 2003).

Mechanisms governing the increase in IGF-1 and the subsequent role played in recovery are unclear. Findings of positive correlation between IGF-1 levels and MMPs 11, 14, TIMPs 1 and 2 as well as stem cell recruitment factor SDF-1 expression, advocate modulation of the ECM and cellular regeneration to be important (Barton et al. 2005; Hall et al. 2004). Clenbuterol treatment of cultured cardiomyocytes has been shown to increase fibroblast-derived IGF-1, causing myocyte hypertrophy via paracrine signalling (Bhavsar et al. 2010; Hall et al. 2004). This suggests that IGF-mediated prevention of myocardial atrophy may also be involved in promoting functional recovery.

3. Clinical aspects of recovery

3.1 Pharmacological enhancement of myocardial recovery

The evidence presented so far suggests that LVAD support can induce significant reverse remodelling in end stage HF, but on its own these changes rarely result in clinical recovery. However, combined pharmacological and LVAD therapy has been shown to achieve greatly improved rates of functional recovery (Birks et al. 2006; Birks et al. 2011) with the greatest rates of explantation being achieved using the Harefield protocol.

3.2 Harefield protocol

A clinical study at Harefield hospital in 2006 achieved an explantation rate of 73% using a novel pharmacological regimen involving the use of the drug clenbuterol, a β_2-AR agonist, in combination with aggressive high dose conventional medical therapy (lisinopril, carvedilol, spironolactone and losartan) (Birks et al. 2006) and pulsatile support. The purpose of this novel treatment strategy, was to enhance LVAD induced myocardial remodelling with high dose "conventional" pharmacotherapy (Phase 1), and prevent LVAD induced myocardial atrophy with high dose (up to 720 mcg tds) clenbuterol (Phase 2). Despite the fact this study was a single centred, small, non-randomised study only involving a small number of patients (n=15), all with non-ischaemic cardiomyopathy, the unprecedented high rates of recovery generated the notion that pharmacological β_2-AR stimulation may enhance myocardial recovery during LVAD therapy, and that future success in making BTR a widespread reality may rest, at least partially upon manipulation of this hitherto overlooked pathway. Support for this rationale has been further strengthened by recent results showing achievement of a 63.2% explantation rate, amongst a DCM cohort (n=20), utilising the same protocol in combination with non-pulsatile mechanical support (Birks et al. 2011).

3.3 Clenbuterol

Clenbuterol is classified as being a selective β_2-AR agent (Baronti et al. 1978) with partial agonist activity, displaying a high affinity for both β_1-ARs and β_2-ARs in a variety of tissues (Cohen et al. 1982). β_2-AR stimulation by various agonists has been shown to cause skeletal muscle hypertrophy in several animal species (Kim et al. 1991). Subsequent results showing clenbuterol to possess a direct "physiological" cardiac hypertrophic effect (Hon et al. 2001) prompted its inclusion in Harefield protocol, primarily as an agent to prevent myocardial atrophy thought to occur with prolonged MU.

3.4 Prevention of myocardial atrophy by clenbuterol

Myocardial atrophy has been widely proposed as one of the mechanisms thwarting myocardial recovery during LVAD treatment of HF, and a plausible explanation for low explantation rates. As part of the Harefield protocol, after stable regression of left ventricular end diastolic dimensions is confirmed echocardiographically over a 2 week period, phase 2 (duration at least 6 mths), consisting of carvedilol being switched to a specific β_1-AR bisoprolol, and the addition of high dose (titrated up to maximum dose of 720 mcg tds) clenbuterol, is commenced.

Lack of echocardiographic measures such as left ventricular posterior wall thickness or relative wall thickness (RWT: interventricular septum thickness + posterior wall thickness/LVEDd), a known predictor of cardiac stability after explantation (Dandel et al. 2008), coupled with the absence of a control group, make it difficult to assess whether "prevention of atrophy" actually occurred in this study. Recovery does not seem to correlate with myocyte size, suggesting that this is not the most important target promoting BTR (Terracciano et al. 2004). Evidence regarding an anti-atrophic action of clenbuterol is equivocal, with experimental studies both supporting (Soppa et al. 2008) as well as opposing (Tsuneyoshi et al. 2005) this effect. A separate small single centre clinical study showed clenbuterol therapy (maximum dose 720mcg od) during MU was effective in preventing cellular atrophy, despite no echocardiographic change in wall thickness (George et al. 2006).

3.5 Other clenbuterol effects

The exact mechanisms through which clenbuterol acts remains unclear, but extensive work undertaken over the last decade, has clearly established that beyond the purely hypertrophic or "anti-atrophic" effects, originally advocating clenbuterol's inclusion in the Harefield protocol, clenbuterol possesses a wide range of other positive actions. Clenbuterol administration for 1 week in normal rats has been shown to cause physiological hypertrophy, increased Ca^{2+} transient amplitude, increased SERCA 2a, PLB, NCX protein levels, and increased SR Ca^{2+} content (Soppa et al. 2005). Clenbuterol (1 week) has also been shown to enhance both whole heart and cellular function in chronically failing rodent myocardium, either alone or in combination with MU , with normalisation of myofilament sensitivity and APD duration and improved NCX activity (Soppa et al. 2008). Increased RyR2, SERCA2a protein expression and decreased apoptosis have been demonstrated in a similar model of HF after long term (9 weeks) clenbuterol therapy (Xydas et al. 2006). In addition, a clear cardioprotective inhibitory G protein dependent anti-apoptotic effect of acute clenbuterol administration has been recently shown during ischaemia reperfusion (Zhang et al. 2010). Clenbuterol modulation of IGF-1 dependent regenerative and hypertrophic pathways, as well as ECM effects may also be responsible for promoting functional recovery (Barton et al. 2005; Bhavsar et al. 2010; Hall et al. 2004).

3.6 Assessment of recovery

3.6.1 Explantation criteria

Echocardiographic, heamodynamic and exercise testing criteria form the foundation on which explantation decisions are made, but specific assessment methods and criteria vary between institutes. At the Berlin Heart Institute LVEF >45%, LVEDd <55mm in the presence of normal central pulmonary pressures, during reduced support (Dandel et al. 2008; Muller et al. 1997) mandates explantation, whereas Harefield hospital employs the criteria of LVEF >45%, LVEDd < 60 mm, LVEDs <50mm, pulmonary capillary wedge pressure <12mm Hg, cardiac index >2.8 l min^{-1} as well as exercise testing criteria, VO_2 max of > 16ml kg^{-1} min^{-1} during "off pump" testing (Birks et al. 2011). Dobutamine stress testing has also been successfully utilised at the Texas Heart Institute (Frazier and Myers 1999).

3.6.2 "Off pump" testing

Off pump testing protocols have been developed relatively recently, and effectively involve cessation of pump flow (> 15 minutes) after systemic heparinisation, followed by assessment of heamodynamic and echocardiographic parameters at rest and after exercise. Turning off of pulsatile devices is acceptable, however turning off non-pulsatile devices leads to retrograde flow across the aortic valve, making functional assessment extremely difficult. This is avoided during testing by decreasing pump speed to 6000 RPM, resulting in zero forward or back flow, effectively ceasing haemodynamic support, or turning the pump "off". Such "off pump" testing has been shown to be safe and well tolerated in both types of device (Birks et al. 2011).

3.6.3 Predictors of recovery

Identification of factors favouring recovery has historically been extremely difficult. Molecular, histological and biochemical markers associated with functional improvement and with recovery have been identified (discussed earlier), but to date no recognised marker is featured in weaning criteria, which remains largely determined by echocardiographic and haemodynamic parameters. Short duration of HF has commonly but not always been shown to favour recovery (Birks et al. 2011), however, recovery of patients with long durations of HF has also been achieved. Echocardiographic parameters at time of LVAD implant are not predictive of recovery, although sustained improvement, as opposed to progressive deterioration in EF, fractional shortening and LV dimensions during LVAD therapy is associated with greater likelihood of explantation (Birks et al. 2011).

3.6.4 Durability of myocardial recovery

The potential therapeutic value of identifying predictors of relapse in preventing LVAD re-implantation has attracted huge interest. Dandel *et al.* identified support duration >6 months, LVEF <45% and LVEDd >55mm at final pre explant echo, as well as a >10% worsening of either of these parameters compared to best obtained value, to be highly predictive of early relapse (Dandel et al. 2008). These findings support the idea that prolonged MU beyond the "optimal point" results in redilatation and functional deterioration (Maybaum et al. 2007). In addition, > 10% decrease in relative wall thickness (RWT: interventricular septum thickness + posterior wall thickness/LVEDd), RWT of <0.38 and duration of HF >5 years, also displayed positive predictive power for post LVAD cardiac instability. Post weaning deterioration in EF and LVEDd within the first 6 months increases risk of HF recurrence, highlighting the importance of early, regular functional surveillance of recovered patients.

3.6.5 Factors opposing recovery

It is proposed that as well as positive remodelling LVADs can induce negative remodelling. Negative remodelling of the ECM, and myocardial atrophy associated with prolonged MU are two potential barriers, thought to be opposing BTR, and pharmacological targeting of these components has yielded some clinical success. Regular and precise functional cardiac assessment during LVAD therapy is essential in promoting BTR. The increasing proportion of new generation devices being implanted as a a means of DT in the US (Kirklin et al. 2011), in which functional recovery is neither expected, promoted, nor assessed may represent a significant new barrier to BTR. Consequently the fraction of LVADs being implanted in the

US as a means of BTR is decreasing (Kirklin et al. 2011) , and a lack of belief in, as well as desire to pursue BTR may mean potentially "recoverable" patients will not be optimised or even assessed for device explantation in the future.

4. Conclusions

Constantly improving technology, the advent of even smaller pumps allowing less traumatic implantation and explantation with fewer complications has already, and will continue to improve LVAD associated morbidity, mortality and quality of life (Rogers et al. 2010). Further use of this unique research vehicle to better understand the reversible mechanisms involved in HF pathogenesis, will identify new therapeutic targets amenable to manipulation. It is probable that if BTR is pursued in future years, recent success suggests it should be (Birks et al. 2006; Birks et al. 2011), combination therapy i.e. LVAD + pharmacotherapy (existing or novel), gene or stem cell therapy, and even a combination of these will yield enhanced rates of recovery. Desires to implant smaller devices in patients with less advanced disease, and implement novel partial unloading, or intermittent ventricular reloading strategies may further improve the BTR strategy and the results of such studies are eagerly awaited.

5. References

Adler, C. P. and Sandritter, W. 1980 Alterations of substances (DNA, myoglobin, myosin, protein) in experimentally induced cardiac hypertrophy and under the influence of drugs (isoproterenol, cytostatics, strophanthin) Basic Res. Cardiol. 75:(1) 126-138

Akgul, A., Skrabal, C. A., Thompson, L. O., Loebe, M., Lafuente, J. A., Noon, G. P., and Youker, K. A. 2004 Role of mast cells and their mediators in failing myocardium under mechanical ventricular support J. Heart Lung Transplant. 23:(6) 709-715

Altemose, G. T., Gritsus, V., Jeevanandam, V., Goldman, B., and Margulies, K. B. 1997 Altered myocardial phenotype after mechanical support in human beings with advanced cardiomyopathy J Heart Lung Transplant. 16:(7) 765-773

Anversa, P. and Kajstura, J. 13-7-1998 Ventricular myocytes are not terminally differentiated in the adult mammalian heart Circ.Res. 83:(1) 1-14

Arnold, J. M., Yusuf, S., Young, J., Mathew, J., Johnstone, D., Avezum, A., Lonn, E., Pogue, J., and Bosch, J. 11-3-2003 Prevention of Heart Failure in Patients in the Heart Outcomes Prevention Evaluation (HOPE) Study Circulation 107:(9) 1284-1290

Ashrafian, H., Frenneaux, M. P., and Opie, L. H. 24-7-2007 Metabolic mechanisms in heart failure Circulation 116:(4) 434-448

Avendano, G. F., Agarwal, R. K., Bashey, R. I., Lyons, M. M., Soni, B. J., Jyothirmayi, G. N., and Regan, T. J. 1999 Effects of glucose intolerance on myocardial function and collagen-linked glycation Diabetes 48:(7) 1443-1447

Baba, H. A., Grabellus, F., August, C., Plenz, G., Takeda, A., Tjan, T. D., Schmid, C., and Deng, M. C. 2000 Reversal of metallothionein expression is different throughout the human myocardium after prolonged left-ventricular mechanical support J.Heart Lung Transplant. 19:(7) 668-674

Badenhorst, D., Maseko, M., Tsotetsi, O. J., Naidoo, A., Brooksbank, R., Norton, G. R., and Woodiwiss, A. J. 2003 Cross-linking influences the impact of quantitative changes in myocardial collagen on cardiac stiffness and remodelling in hypertension in rats Cardiovasc.Res. 57:(3) 632-641

Baronti, A., Griceo, A., and Vibelli, C. 31-5-1978 Study of a new oral beta-adrenergic drug, clenbuterol, in patients with chronic bronchitis Eur.J.Clin.Pharmacol. 13:(3) 171-177

Bartha, E., Kiss, G. N., Kalman, E., Kulcsar, G., Kalai, T., Hideg, K., Habon, T., Sumegi, B., Toth, K., and Halmosi, R. 2008 Effect of L-2286, a poly(ADP-ribose)polymerase inhibitor and enalapril on myocardial remodeling and heart failure J.Cardiovasc.Pharmacol. 52:(3) 253-261

Bartling, B., Milting, H., Schumann, H., Darmer, D., Arusoglu, L., Koerner, M. M., El-Banayosy, A., Koerfer, R., Holtz, J., and Zerkowski, H. R. 9-11-1999 Myocardial gene expression of regulators of myocyte apoptosis and myocyte calcium homeostasis during hemodynamic unloading by ventricular assist devices in patients with end-stage heart failure Circulation 100:(19 Suppl) II216-II223

Barton, P. J., Felkin, L. E., Birks, E. J., Cullen, M. E., Banner, N. R., Grindle, S., Hall, J. L., Miller, L. W., and Yacoub, M. H. 30-8-2005 Myocardial insulin-like growth factor-I gene expression during recovery from heart failure after combined left ventricular assist device and clenbuterol therapy Circulation 112:(9 Suppl) I46-I50

Beltrami, A. P., Urbanek, K., Kajstura, J., Yan, S. M., Finato, N., Bussani, R., Nadal-Ginard, B., Silvestri, F., Leri, A., Beltrami, C. A., and Anversa, P. 7-6-2001 Evidence that human cardiac myocytes divide after myocardial infarction N. Engl. J. Med. 344:(23) 1750-1757

Bers, D. M. 2006 Altered cardiac myocyte Ca regulation in heart failure Physiology. (Bethesda.) 21:() 380-387

Bhavsar, P. K., Brand, N. J., Felkin, L. E., Luther, P. K., Cullen, M. E., Yacoub, M. H., and Barton, P. J. 2010 Clenbuterol induces cardiac myocyte hypertrophy via paracrine signalling and fibroblast-derived IGF-1 J. Cardiovasc. Transl. Res. 3:(6) 688-695

Birks, E. J., George, R. S., Hedger, M., Bahrami, T., Wilton, P., Bowles, C. T., Webb, C., Bougard, R., Amrani, M., Yacoub, M. H., Dreyfus, G., and Khaghani, A. 1-2-2011 Reversal of severe heart failure with a continuous-flow left ventricular assist device and pharmacological therapy: a prospective study Circulation 123:(4) 381-390

Birks, E. J., Hall, J. L., Barton, P. J., Grindle, S., Latif, N., Hardy, J. P., Rider, J. E., Banner, N. R., Khaghani, A., Miller, L. W., and Yacoub, M. H. 30-8-2005 Gene profiling changes in cytoskeletal proteins during clinical recovery after left ventricular-assist device support Circulation 112:(9 Suppl) I57-I64

Birks, E. J., Latif, N., Owen, V., Bowles, C., Felkin, L. E., Mullen, A. J., Khaghani, A., Barton, P. J., Polak, J. M., Pepper, J. R., Banner, N. R., and Yacoub, M. H. 18-9-2001 Quantitative myocardial cytokine expression and activation of the apoptotic pathway in patients who require left ventricular assist devices Circulation 104:(12 Suppl 1) I233-I240

Birks, E. J., Tansley, P. D., Hardy, J., George, R. S., Bowles, C. T., Burke, M., Banner, N. R., Khaghani, A., and Yacoub, M. H. 2-11-2006 Left ventricular assist device and drug therapy for the reversal of heart failure N. Engl. J Med. 355:(18) 1873-1884

Bonnefont-Rousselot, D., Mahmoudi, A., Mougenot, N., Varoquaux, O., Le, Nahour G., Fouret, P., and Lechat, P. 2002 Catecholamine effects on cardiac remodelling, oxidative stress and fibrosis in experimental heart failure Redox. Rep. 7:(3) 145-151

Bouchard, R. A., Clark, R. B., and Giles, W. R. 1995 Effects of action potential duration on excitation-contraction coupling in rat ventricular myocytes. Action potential voltage-clamp measurements Circ. Res. 76:(5) 790-801

Bruckner, B. A., Stetson, S. J., Farmer, J. A., Radovancevic, B., Frazier, O. H., Noon, G. P., Entman, M. L., Torre-Amione, G., and Youker, K. A. 2000 The implications for cardiac recovery of left ventricular assist device support on myocardial collagen content Am J Surg. 180:(6) 498-501

Bruckner, B. A., Stetson, S. J., Perez-Verdia, A., Youker, K. A., Radovancevic, B., Connelly, J. H., Koerner, M. M., Entman, M. E., Frazier, O. H., Noon, G. P., and Torre-Amione, G. 2001 Regression of fibrosis and hypertrophy in failing myocardium following mechanical circulatory support J Heart Lung Transplant. 20:(4) 457-464

Bruggink, A. H., van Oosterhout, M. F., De, Jonge N., Ivangh, B., van, Kuik J., Voorbij, R. H., Cleutjens, J. P., Gmelig-Meyling, F. H., and De Weger, R. A. 2006 Reverse remodeling of the myocardial extracellular matrix after prolonged left ventricular assist device support follows a biphasic pattern J Heart Lung Transplant. 25:(9) 1091-1098

Busk, P. K., Bartkova, J., Strom, C. C., Wulf-Andersen, L., Hinrichsen, R., Christoffersen, T. E., Latella, L., Bartek, J., Haunso, S., and Sheikh, S. P. 2002 Involvement of cyclin D activity in left ventricle hypertrophy in vivo and in vitro Cardiovasc. Res. 56:(1) 64-75

Chaudhary, K. W., Rossman, E. I., Piacentino, V., III, Kenessey, A., Weber, C., Gaughan, J. P., Ojamaa, K., Klein, I., Bers, D. M., Houser, S. R., and Margulies, K. B. 18-8-2004 Altered myocardial Ca2+ cycling after left ventricular assist device support in the failing human heart J Am Coll.Cardiol. 44:(4) 837-845

Cohen, M. L., Wiley, K. S., and Bemis, K. G. 1982 Analysis of the beta 1 and beta 2 adrenoceptor interactions of the partial agonist, clenbuterol (NAB365), in the rat jugular vein and atria Naunyn Schmiedebergs Arch.Pharmacol. 320:(2) 145-151

Cohn, J. N. 15-8-1996 The management of chronic heart failure N.Engl.J.Med. 335:(7) 490-498

Dandel, M., Weng, Y., Siniawski, H., Potapov, E., Drews, T., Lehmkuhl, H. B., Knosalla, C., and Hetzer, R. 30-9-2008 Prediction of cardiac stability after weaning from left ventricular assist devices in patients with idiopathic dilated cardiomyopathy 17 Circulation 118:(14 Suppl) S94-105

Dandel, M., Weng, Y., Siniawski, H., Potapov, E., Lehmkuhl, H. B., and Hetzer, R. 30-8-2005 Long-term results in patients with idiopathic dilated cardiomyopathy after weaning from left ventricular assist devices Circulation 112:(9 Suppl) I37-I45

De, Jonge N., van Wichen, D. F., Schipper, M. E., Lahpor, J. R., Gmelig-Meyling, F. H., Robles de Medina, E. O., and De Weger, R. A. 20-3-2002 Left ventricular assist device in end-stage heart failure: persistence of structural myocyte damage after unloading. An immunohistochemical analysis of the contractile myofilaments J.Am.Coll.Cardiol. 39:(6) 963-969

Delgado, R., III, Radovancevic, B., Massin, E. K., Frazier, O. H., and Benedict, C. 1998 Neurohormonal changes after implantation of a left ventricular assist system ASAIO J. 44:(4) 299-302

Dipla, K., Mattiello, J. A., Jeevanandam, V., Houser, S. R., and Margulies, K. B. 16-6-1998 Myocyte recovery after mechanical circulatory support in humans with end-stage heart failure Circulation 97:(23) 2316-2322

Duerr, R. L., Huang, S., Miraliakbar, H. R., Clark, R., Chien, K. R., and Ross, J., Jr. 1995 Insulin-like growth factor-1 enhances ventricular hypertrophy and function during the onset of experimental cardiac failure J.Clin.Invest 95:(2) 619-627

Duerr, R. L., McKirnan, M. D., Gim, R. D., Clark, R. G., Chien, K. R., and Ross, J., Jr. 15-6-1996 Cardiovascular effects of insulin-like growth factor-1 and growth hormone in chronic left ventricular failure in the rat Circulation 93:(12) 2188-2196

Engel, F. B., Hsieh, P. C., Lee, R. T., and Keating, M. T. 17-10-2006 FGF1/p38 MAP kinase inhibitor therapy induces cardiomyocyte mitosis, reduces scarring, and rescues function after myocardial infarction Proc.Natl.Acad.Sci.U.S.A 103:(42) 15546-15551

Farrar, D. J., Holman, W. R., McBride, L. R., Kormos, R. L., Icenogle, T. B., Hendry, P. J., Moore, C. H., Loisance, D. Y., El-Banayosy, A., and Frazier, H. 2002 Long-term follow-up of Thoratec ventricular assist device bridge-to-recovery patients successfully removed from support after recovery of ventricular function J.Heart Lung Transplant. 21:(5) 516-521

Felkin, L. E., Lara-Pezzi, E., George, R., Yacoub, M. H., Birks, E. J., and Barton, P. J. 2009 Expression of extracellular matrix genes during myocardial recovery from heart failure after left ventricular assist device support J.Heart Lung Transplant. 28:(2) 117-122

Francis, G. S., Anwar, F., Bank, A. J., Kubo, S. H., and Jessurun, J. 1999 Apoptosis, Bcl-2, and proliferating cell nuclear antigen in the failing human heart: observations made after implantation of left ventricular assist device J.Card Fail. 5:(4) 308-315

Frazier, O. H. 1994 First use of an untethered, vented electric left ventricular assist device for long-term support Circulation 89:(6) 2908-2914

Frazier, O. H., Benedict, C. R., Radovancevic, B., Bick, R. J., Capek, P., Springer, W. E., Macris, M. P., Delgado, R., and Buja, L. M. 1996 Improved left ventricular function after chronic left ventricular unloading 1 Ann.Thorac.Surg. 62:(3) 675-681

Frazier, O. H. and Myers, T. J. 1999 Left ventricular assist system as a bridge to myocardial recovery Ann.Thorac.Surg. 68:(2) 734-741

Gaughan, J. P., Furukawa, S., Jeevanandam, V., Hefner, C. A., Kubo, H., Margulies, K. B., McGowan, B. S., Mattiello, J. A., Dipla, K., Piacentino, V., III, Li, S., and Houser, S. R. 1999 Sodium/calcium exchange contributes to contraction and relaxation in failed human ventricular myocytes Am.J.Physiol 277:(2 Pt 2) H714-H724

George, I., Xydas, S., Mancini, D. M., LaManca, J., DiTullio, M., Marboe, C. C., Shane, E., Schulman, A. R., Colley, P. M., Petrilli, C. M., Naka, Y., Oz, M. C., and Maybaum, S. 2006 Effect of clenbuterol on cardiac and skeletal muscle function during left ventricular assist device support 8 J.Heart Lung Transplant. 25:(9) 1084-1090

Gwathmey, J. K., Copelas, L., MacKinnon, R., Schoen, F. J., Feldman, M. D., Grossman, W., and Morgan, J. P. 1987 Abnormal intracellular calcium handling in myocardium from patients with end-stage heart failure Circ.Res. 61:(1) 70-76

Hall, J. L., Birks, E. J., Grindle, S., Cullen, M. E., Barton, P. J., Rider, J. E., Lee, S., Harwalker, S., Mariash, A., Adhikari, N., Charles, N. J., Felkin, L. E., Polster, S., George, R. S., Miller, L. W., and Yacoub, M. H. 2007 Molecular signature of recovery following combination left ventricular assist device (LVAD) support and pharmacologic therapy Eur.Heart J. 28:(5) 613-627

Hall, J. L., Grindle, S., Han, X., Fermin, D., Park, S., Chen, Y., Bache, R. J., Mariash, A., Guan, Z., Ormaza, S., Thompson, J., Graziano, J., de Sam Lazaro, S. E., Pan, S., Simari, R. D., and Miller, L. W. 19-5-2004 Genomic profiling of the human heart before and after mechanical support with a ventricular assist device reveals alterations in vascular signaling networks Physiol Genomics 17:(3) 283-291

Harding, J. D., Piacentino, V., III, Gaughan, J. P., Houser, S. R., and Margulies, K. B. 11-9-2001 Electrophysiological alterations after mechanical circulatory support in patients with advanced cardiac failure Circulation 104:(11) 1241-1247

Hasenfuss, G., Schillinger, W., Lehnart, S. E., Preuss, M., Pieske, B., Maier, L. S., Prestle, J., Minami, K., and Just, H. 9-2-1999 Relationship between Na+-Ca2+-exchanger protein levels and diastolic function of failing human myocardium Circulation 99:(5) 641-648

Heerdt, P. M., Holmes, J. W., Cai, B., Barbone, A., Madigan, J. D., Reiken, S., Lee, D. L., Oz, M. C., Marks, A. R., and Burkhoff, D. 28-11-2000a Chronic unloading by left ventricular assist device reverses contractile dysfunction and alters gene expression in end-stage heart failure Circulation 102:(22) 2713-2719

Heerdt, P. M., Holmes, J. W., Cai, B., Barbone, A., Madigan, J. D., Reiken, S., Lee, D. L., Oz, M. C., Marks, A. R., and Burkhoff, D. 28-11-2000b Chronic unloading by left ventricular assist device reverses contractile dysfunction and alters gene expression in end-stage heart failure Circulation 102:(22) 2713-2719

Heerdt, P. M., Schlame, M., Jehle, R., Barbone, A., Burkhoff, D., and Blanck, T. J. 2002 Disease-specific remodeling of cardiac mitochondria after a left ventricular assist device Ann.Thorac.Surg. 73:(4) 1216-1221

Hetzer, R., Muller, J. H., Weng, Y. G., Loebe, M., and Wallukat, G. 2000 Midterm follow-up of patients who underwent removal of a left ventricular assist device after cardiac recovery from end-stage dilated cardiomyopathy J Thorac.Cardiovasc.Surg. 120:(5) 843-853

Hon, J. K., Steendijk, P., Petrou, M., Wong, K., and Yacoub, M. H. 2001 Influence of clenbuterol treatment during six weeks of chronic right ventricular pressure overload as studied with pressure-volume analysis 21 J.Thorac.Cardiovasc.Surg. 122:(4) 767-774

Hosoda, T., Kajstura, J., Leri, A., and Anversa, P. 2010 Mechanisms of myocardial regeneration Circ.J. 74:(1) 13-17

Hubler, S., Potapov, E. V., Loebe, M., Nasseri, B. A., Gosmann, D., Hoffmann, K., Sodian, R., Hausmann, H., and Hetzer, R. 2003 Development of a database of patients supported by ventricular assist devices ASAIO J. 49:(3) 340-344

Hunt, S. A., Abraham, W. T., Chin, M. H., Feldman, A. M., Francis, G. S., Ganiats, T. G., Jessup, M., Konstam, M. A., Mancini, D. M., Michl, K., Oates, J. A., Rahko, P. S., Silver, M. A., Stevenson, L. W., and Yancy, C. W. 14-4-2009a 2009 Focused update incorporated into the ACC/AHA 2005 Guidelines for the Diagnosis and Management of Heart Failure in Adults A Report of the American College of Cardiology Foundation/American Heart Association Task Force on Practice Guidelines Developed in Collaboration With the International Society for Heart and Lung Transplantation J.Am.Coll.Cardiol. 53:(15) e1-e90

Hunt, S. A., Abraham, W. T., Chin, M. H., Feldman, A. M., Francis, G. S., Ganiats, T. G., Jessup, M., Konstam, M. A., Mancini, D. M., Michl, K., Oates, J. A., Rahko, P. S., Silver, M. A., Stevenson, L. W., and Yancy, C. W. 14-4-2009b 2009 focused update incorporated into the ACC/AHA 2005 Guidelines for the Diagnosis and Management of Heart Failure in Adults: a report of the American College of Cardiology Foundation/American Heart Association Task Force on Practice Guidelines: developed in collaboration with the International Society for Heart and Lung Transplantation Circulation 119:(14) e391-e479

Ibrahim, M. A., Ashour, O. M., Ibrahim, Y. F., El-Bitar, H. I., Gomaa, W., and bdel-Rahim, S. R. 2009 Angiotensin-converting enzyme inhibition and angiotensin AT(1)-receptor antagonism equally improve doxorubicin-induced cardiotoxicity and nephrotoxicity Pharmacol.Res. 60:(5) 373-381

Ingwall, J. S. and Weiss, R. G. 23-7-2004 Is the failing heart energy starved? On using chemical energy to support cardiac function Circ.Res. 95:(2) 135-145

Jessup, M. and Brozena, S. 15-5-2003 Heart failure N.Engl.J.Med. 348:(20) 2007-2018

Kim, Y. S., Sainz, R. D., Molenaar, P., and Summers, R. J. 9-10-1991 Characterization of beta 1- and beta 2-adrenoceptors in rat skeletal muscles 1 Biochem.Pharmacol. 42:(9) 1783-1789

Kirklin, J. K., Naftel, D. C., Kormos, R. L., Stevenson, L. W., Pagani, F. D., Miller, M. A., Ulisney, K. L., Baldwin, J. T., and Young, J. B. 2011 Third INTERMACS Annual Report: the evolution of destination therapy in the United States J.Heart Lung Transplant. 30:(2) 115-123

Klotz, S., Barbone, A., Reiken, S., Holmes, J. W., Naka, Y., Oz, M. C., Marks, A. R., and Burkhoff, D. 1-3-2005a Left ventricular assist device support normalizes left and right ventricular beta-adrenergic pathway properties J.Am.Coll.Cardiol. 45:(5) 668-676

Klotz, S., Burkhoff, D., Garrelds, I. M., Boomsma, F., and Danser, A. H. 2009 The impact of left ventricular assist device-induced left ventricular unloading on the myocardial renin-angiotensin-aldosterone system: therapeutic consequences? Eur.Heart J. 30:(7) 805-812

Klotz, S., Danser, A. H., Foronjy, R. F., Oz, M. C., Wang, J., Mancini, D., D'Armiento, J., and Burkhoff, D. 20-3-2007a The impact of angiotensin-converting enzyme inhibitor therapy on the extracellular collagen matrix during left ventricular assist device support in patients with end-stage heart failure J Am Coll.Cardiol. 49:(11) 1166-1174

Klotz, S., Danser, A. H., Foronjy, R. F., Oz, M. C., Wang, J., Mancini, D., D'Armiento, J., and Burkhoff, D. 20-3-2007b The impact of angiotensin-converting enzyme inhibitor therapy on the extracellular collagen matrix during left ventricular assist device support in patients with end-stage heart failure J Am Coll.Cardiol. 49:(11) 1166-1174

Klotz, S., Foronjy, R. F., Dickstein, M. L., Gu, A., Garrelds, I. M., Danser, A. H., Oz, M. C., D'Armiento, J., and Burkhoff, D. 19-7-2005b Mechanical unloading during left ventricular assist device support increases left ventricular collagen cross-linking and myocardial stiffness Circulation 112:(3) 364-374

Klotz, S., Jan Danser, A. H., and Burkhoff, D. 2008 Impact of left ventricular assist device (LVAD) support on the cardiac reverse remodeling process Prog.Biophys.Mol.Biol. 97:(2-3) 479-496

Komuro, I., Wenninger, K. E., Philipson, K. D., and Izumo, S. 15-5-1992 Molecular cloning and characterization of the human cardiac Na+/Ca2+ exchanger cDNA Proc.Natl.Acad.Sci.U.S.A 89:(10) 4769-4773

Koss, K. L., Grupp, I. L., and Kranias, E. G. 1997 The relative phospholamban and SERCA2 ratio: a critical determinant of myocardial contractility Basic Res.Cardiol. 92 Suppl 1:() 17-24

Kuhn, M., Voss, M., Mitko, D., Stypmann, J., Schmid, C., Kawaguchi, N., Grabellus, F., and Baba, H. A. 1-11-2004 Left ventricular assist device support reverses altered cardiac expression and function of natriuretic peptides and receptors in end-stage heart failure Cardiovasc.Res. 64:(2) 308-314

Kushnir, A. and Marks, A. R. 2010 The ryanodine receptor in cardiac physiology and disease Adv.Pharmacol. 59:() 1-30

Latif, N., Yacoub, M. H., George, R., Barton, P. J., and Birks, E. J. 2007 Changes in sarcomeric and non-sarcomeric cytoskeletal proteins and focal adhesion molecules during clinical myocardial recovery after left ventricular assist device support J.Heart Lung Transplant. 26:(3) 230-235

Lee, S. H., Doliba, N., Osbakken, M., Oz, M., and Mancini, D. 1998 Improvement of myocardial mitochondrial function after hemodynamic support with left ventricular assist devices in patients with heart failure J.Thorac.Cardiovasc.Surg. 116:(2) 344-349

Leri, A., Kajstura, J., and Anversa, P. 2005 Cardiac stem cells and mechanisms of myocardial regeneration Physiol Rev. 85:(4) 1373-1416

Levin, H. R., Oz, M. C., Chen, J. M., Packer, M., Rose, E. A., and Burkhoff, D. 1-6-1995 Reversal of chronic ventricular dilation in patients with end-stage cardiomyopathy by prolonged mechanical unloading Circulation 91:(11) 2717-2720

Li, Q., Li, B., Wang, X., Leri, A., Jana, K. P., Liu, Y., Kajstura, J., Baserga, R., and Anversa, P. 15-10-1997 Overexpression of insulin-like growth factor-1 in mice protects from myocyte death after infarction, attenuating ventricular dilation, wall stress, and cardiac hypertrophy J.Clin.Invest 100:(8) 1991-1999

Li, Y. Y., Feng, Y., McTiernan, C. F., Pei, W., Moravec, C. S., Wang, P., Rosenblum, W., Kormos, R. L., and Feldman, A. M. 4-9-2001 Downregulation of matrix metalloproteinases and reduction in collagen damage in the failing human heart after support with left ventricular assist devices Circulation 104:(10) 1147-1152

Madigan, J. D., Barbone, A., Choudhri, A. F., Morales, D. L., Cai, B., Oz, M. C., and Burkhoff, D. 2001 Time course of reverse remodeling of the left ventricle during support with a left ventricular assist device J.Thorac.Cardiovasc.Surg. 121:(5) 902-908

Mancini, D. and Lietz, K. 13-7-2010 Selection of cardiac transplantation candidates in 2010 Circulation 122:(2) 173-183

Mann, D. L. and Spinale, F. G. 27-10-1998 Activation of matrix metalloproteinases in the failing human heart: breaking the tie that binds Circulation 98:(17) 1699-1702

Marijianowski, M. M., Teeling, P., Mann, J., and Becker, A. E. 1995 Dilated cardiomyopathy is associated with an increase in the type I/type III collagen ratio: a quantitative assessment J.Am.Coll.Cardiol. 25:(6) 1263-1272

Marx, S. O., Reiken, S., Hisamatsu, Y., Jayaraman, T., Burkhoff, D., Rosemblit, N., and Marks, A. R. 12-5-2000 PKA phosphorylation dissociates FKBP12.6 from the calcium release channel (ryanodine receptor): defective regulation in failing hearts Cell 101:(4) 365-376

Matsumiya, G., Monta, O., Fukushima, N., Sawa, Y., Funatsu, T., Toda, K., and Matsuda, H. 2005 Who would be a candidate for bridge to recovery during prolonged mechanical left ventricular support in idiopathic dilated cardiomyopathy? J.Thorac.Cardiovasc.Surg. 130:(3) 699-704

Maybaum, S., Kamalakannan, G., and Murthy, S. 2008 Cardiac recovery during mechanical assist device support Semin.Thorac.Cardiovasc.Surg. 20:(3) 234-246

Maybaum, S., Mancini, D., Xydas, S., Starling, R. C., Aaronson, K., Pagani, F. D., Miller, L. W., Margulies, K., McRee, S., Frazier, O. H., and Torre-Amione, G. 15-5-2007 Cardiac improvement during mechanical circulatory support: a prospective multicenter study of the LVAD Working Group Circulation 115:(19) 2497-2505

Mayosi, B. M. 2007 Contemporary trends in the epidemiology and management of cardiomyopathy and pericarditis in sub-Saharan Africa Heart 93:(10) 1176-1183

McCarthy, P. M., Savage, R. M., Fraser, C. D., Vargo, R., James, K. B., Goormastic, M., and Hobbs, R. E. 1995 Hemodynamic and physiologic changes during support with an implantable left ventricular assist device J Thorac.Cardiovasc.Surg. 109:(3) 409-417

Mehta, S. M., Aufiero, T. X., Pae, W. E., Jr., Miller, C. A., and Pierce, W. S. 1996 Results of mechanical ventricular assistance for the treatment of post cardiotomy cardiogenic shock ASAIO J. 42:(3) 211-218

Meng, G., Wu, F., Yang, L., Zhu, H., Gu, J., He, M., and Xu, J. 2009 Synergistic attenuation of myocardial fibrosis in spontaneously hypertensive rats by joint treatment with benazepril and candesartan J.Cardiovasc.Pharmacol. 54:(1) 16-24

Milting, H., Bartling, B., Schumann, H., El-Banayosy, A., Wlost, S., Ruter, F., Darmer, D., Holtz, J., Korfer, R., and Zerkowski, H. R. 1999 Altered levels of mRNA of apoptosis-mediating genes after mid-term mechanical ventricular support in dilative cardiomyopathy--first results of the Halle Assist Induced Recovery Study (HAIR) Thorac.Cardiovasc.Surg. 47:(1) 48-50

Milting, H., Scholz, C., Arusoglu, L., Freitag, M., Cebulla, R., Jaquet, K., Korfer, R., Lewinski, V., Kassner, A., Brodde, O. E., Kogler, H., El, Banayosy A., and Pieske, B. 2006 Selective upregulation of beta1-adrenergic receptors and dephosphorylation of troponin I in end-stage heart failure patients supported by ventricular assist devices J.Mol.Cell Cardiol. 41:(3) 441-450

Mohapatra, B., Vick, G. W., III, Fraser, C. D., Jr., Clunie, S. K., Towbin, J. A., Sinagra, G., and Vatta, M. 2010 Short-term mechanical unloading and reverse remodeling of failing hearts in children J.Heart Lung Transplant. 29:(1) 98-104

Mukherjee, D. and Sen, S. 1991 Alteration of collagen phenotypes in ischemic cardiomyopathy J.Clin.Invest 88:(4) 1141-1146

Muller, J., Wallukat, G., Weng, Y. G., Dandel, M., Spiegelsberger, S., Semrau, S., Brandes, K., Theodoridis, V., Loebe, M., Meyer, R., and Hetzer, R. 15-7-1997 Weaning from mechanical cardiac support in patients with idiopathic dilated cardiomyopathy Circulation 96:(2) 542-549

Musaro, A. 2005 Growth factor enhancement of muscle regeneration: a central role of IGF-1 Arch.Ital.Biol. 143:(3-4) 243-248

Narula, J., Haider, N., Arbustini, E., and Chandrashekhar, Y. 2006 Mechanisms of disease: apoptosis in heart failure--seeing hope in death Nat.Clin.Pract.Cardiovasc.Med. 3:(12) 681-688

Neubauer, S. 15-3-2007 The failing heart--an engine out of fuel N.Engl.J.Med. 356:(11) 1140-1151

Ogletree, M. L., Sweet, W. E., Talerico, C., Klecka, M. E., Young, J. B., Smedira, N. G., Starling, R. C., and Moravec, C. S. 2010 Duration of left ventricular assist device support: Effects on abnormal calcium cycling and functional recovery in the failing human heart J.Heart Lung Transplant. 29:(5) 554-561

Ogletree-Hughes, M. L., Stull, L. B., Sweet, W. E., Smedira, N. G., McCarthy, P. M., and Moravec, C. S. 21-8-2001 Mechanical unloading restores beta-adrenergic responsiveness and reverses receptor downregulation in the failing human heart Circulation 104:(8) 881-886

Oriyanhan, W., Tsuneyoshi, H., Nishina, T., Matsuoka, S., Ikeda, T., and Komeda, M. 2007 Determination of optimal duration of mechanical unloading for failing hearts to achieve bridge to recovery in a rat heterotopic heart transplantation model J Heart Lung Transplant. 26:(1) 16-23

Pelosi, L., Giacinti, C., Nardis, C., Borsellino, G., Rizzuto, E., Nicoletti, C., Wannenes, F., Battistini, L., Rosenthal, N., Molinaro, M., and Musaro, A. 2007 Local expression of IGF-1 accelerates muscle regeneration by rapidly modulating inflammatory cytokines and chemokines FASEB J. 21:(7) 1393-1402

Pieske, B., Sutterlin, M., Schmidt-Schweda, S., Minami, K., Meyer, M., Olschewski, M., Holubarsch, C., Just, H., and Hasenfuss, G. 1-8-1996 Diminished post-rest potentiation of contractile force in human dilated cardiomyopathy. Functional evidence for alterations in intracellular Ca2+ handling J.Clin.Invest 98:(3) 764-776

Porter, K. E. and Turner, N. A. 2009 Cardiac fibroblasts: at the heart of myocardial remodeling Pharmacol.Ther. 123:(2) 255-278

Razeghi, P., Bruckner, B. A., Sharma, S., Youker, K. A., Frazier, O. H., and Taegtmeyer, H. 2003 Mechanical unloading of the failing human heart fails to activate the protein kinase B/Akt/glycogen synthase kinase-3beta survival pathway Cardiology 100:(1) 17-22

Razeghi, P., Mukhopadhyay, M., Myers, T. J., Williams, J. N., Moravec, C. S., Frazier, O. H., and Taegtmeyer, H. 2001 Myocardial tumor necrosis factor-alpha expression does not correlate with clinical indices of heart failure in patients on left ventricular assist device support Ann.Thorac.Surg. 72:(6) 2044-2050

Rogers, J. G., Aaronson, K. D., Boyle, A. J., Russell, S. D., Milano, C. A., Pagani, F. D., Edwards, B. S., Park, S., John, R., Conte, J. V., Farrar, D. J., and Slaughter, M. S. 27-4-2010 Continuous flow left ventricular assist device improves functional capacity and quality of life of advanced heart failure patients J.Am.Coll.Cardiol. 55:(17) 1826-1834

Saito, S., Matsumiya, G., Sakaguchi, T., Miyagawa, S., Yamauchi, T., Kuratani, T., and Sawa, Y. 2010 Cardiac fibrosis and cellular hypertrophy decrease the degree of reverse remodeling and improvement in cardiac function during left ventricular assist J.Heart Lung Transplant. 29:(6) 672-679

Sandritter, W. and Adler, C. P. 26-5-1976 Polyploidization of heart muscle nuclei as a prerequisite for heart growth and numerical hyperplasia in heart hypertrophy Recent Adv.Stud.Cardiac.Struct.Metab 12:() 115-127

Santini, M. P., Tsao, L., Monassier, L., Theodoropoulos, C., Carter, J., Lara-Pezzi, E., Slonimsky, E., Salimova, E., Delafontaine, P., Song, Y. H., Bergmann, M., Freund, C., Suzuki, K., and Rosenthal, N. 22-6-2007 Enhancing repair of the mammalian heart Circ.Res. 100:(12) 1732-1740

Shahar, E., Lee, S., Kim, J., Duval, S., Barber, C., and Luepker, R. V. 2004 Hospitalized heart failure: rates and long-term mortality J.Card Fail. 10:(5) 374-379

Shan, J., Betzenhauser, M. J., Kushnir, A., Reiken, S., Meli, A. C., Wronska, A., Dura, M., Chen, B. X., and Marks, A. R. 1-12-2010 Role of chronic ryanodine receptor phosphorylation in heart failure and beta-adrenergic receptor blockade in mice J.Clin.Invest 120:(12) 4375-4387

Simon, M. A., Kormos, R. L., Murali, S., Nair, P., Heffernan, M., Gorcsan, J., Winowich, S., and McNamara, D. M. 30-8-2005 Myocardial recovery using ventricular assist devices: prevalence, clinical characteristics, and outcomes Circulation 112:(9 Suppl) I32-I36

Soppa, G. K., Lee, J., Stagg, M. A., Felkin, L. E., Barton, P. J., Siedlecka, U., Youssef, S., Yacoub, M. H., and Terracciano, C. M. 1-3-2008 Role and possible mechanisms of clenbuterol in enhancing reverse remodelling during mechanical unloading in murine heart failure Cardiovasc.Res 77:(4) 695-706

Soppa, G. K., Smolenski, R. T., Latif, N., Yuen, A. H., Malik, A., Karbowska, J., Kochan, Z., Terracciano, C. M., and Yacoub, M. H. 2005 Effects of chronic administration of clenbuterol on function and metabolism of adult rat cardiac muscle Am J Physiol Heart Circ Physiol 288:(3) H1468-H1476

Spinale, F. G., Coker, M. L., Heung, L. J., Bond, B. R., Gunasinghe, H. R., Etoh, T., Goldberg, A. T., Zellner, J. L., and Crumbley, A. J. 17-10-2000 A matrix metalloproteinase induction/activation system exists in the human left ventricular myocardium and is upregulated in heart failure Circulation 102:(16) 1944-1949

Starling, R. C., Hammer, D. F., and Altschuld, R. A. 1998 Human myocardial ATP content and in vivo contractile function Mol.Cell Biochem. 180:(1-2) 171-177

Sylvin, E. A., Stern, D. R., and Goldstein, D. J. 2010 Mechanical support for postcardiotomy cardiogenic shock: has progress been made? J.Card Surg. 25:(4) 442-454

Takaseya, T., Ishimatsu, M., Tayama, E., Nishi, A., Akasu, T., and Aoyagi, S. 7-12-2004 Mechanical unloading improves intracellular Ca2+ regulation in rats with doxorubicin-induced cardiomyopathy J Am Coll.Cardiol. 44:(11) 2239-2246

Terracciano, C. M., Hardy, J., Birks, E. J., Khaghani, A., Banner, N. R., and Yacoub, M. H. 18-5-2004 Clinical recovery from end-stage heart failure using left-ventricular assist device and pharmacological therapy correlates with increased sarcoplasmic reticulum calcium content but not with regression of cellular hypertrophy Circulation 109:(19) 2263-2265

Terracciano, C. M., Koban, M. U., Soppa, G. K., Siedlecka, U., Lee, J., Stagg, M. A., and Yacoub, M. H. 2007 The role of the cardiac Na+/Ca2+ exchanger in reverse remodeling: relevance for LVAD-recovery Ann.N.Y.Acad.Sci. 1099:() 349-360

Terracciano, C. M., Miller, L. W., and Yacoub, M. H. 2010 Contemporary use of ventricular assist devices Annu.Rev.Med. 61:() 255-270

Thohan, V., Stetson, S. J., Nagueh, S. F., Rivas-Gotz, C., Koerner, M. M., Lafuente, J. A., Loebe, M., Noon, G. P., and Torre-Amione, G. 2005 Cellular and hemodynamics responses of failing myocardium to continuous flow mechanical circulatory support using the DeBakey-Noon left ventricular assist device: a comparative analysis with pulsatile-type devices J.Heart Lung Transplant. 24:(5) 566-575

Thompson, L. O., Skrabal, C. A., Loebe, M., Lafuente, J. A., Roberts, R. R., Akgul, A., Jones, V., Bruckner, B. A., Thohan, V., Noon, G. P., and Youker, K. A. 2005 Plasma neurohormone levels correlate with left ventricular functional and morphological improvement in LVAD patients J.Surg.Res. 123:(1) 25-32

Torre-Amione, G., Stetson, S. J., Youker, K. A., Durand, J. B., Radovancevic, B., Delgado, R. M., Frazier, O. H., Entman, M. L., and Noon, G. P. 14-9-1999 Decreased expression of tumor necrosis factor-alpha in failing human myocardium after mechanical circulatory support : A potential mechanism for cardiac recovery Circulation 100:(11) 1189-1193

Trulock, E. P., Christie, J. D., Edwards, L. B., Boucek, M. M., Aurora, P., Taylor, D. O., Dobbels, F., Rahmel, A. O., Keck, B. M., and Hertz, M. I. 2007 Registry of the International Society for Heart and Lung Transplantation: twenty-fourth official adult lung and heart-lung transplantation report-2007 J.Heart Lung Transplant. 26:(8) 782-795

Tsuneyoshi, H., Oriyanhan, W., Kanemitsu, H., Shiina, R., Nishina, T., Matsuoka, S., Ikeda, T., and Komeda, M. 30-8-2005 Does the beta2-agonist clenbuterol help to maintain myocardial potential to recover during mechanical unloading? 1 Circulation 112:(9 Suppl) I51-I56

Urbanek, K., Torella, D., Sheikh, F., De, Angelis A., Nurzynska, D., Silvestri, F., Beltrami, C. A., Bussani, R., Beltrami, A. P., Quaini, F., Bolli, R., Leri, A., Kajstura, J., and Anversa, P. 14-6-2005 Myocardial regeneration by activation of multipotent cardiac stem cells in ischemic heart failure Proc.Natl.Acad.Sci.U.S.A 102:(24) 8692-8697

Vatta, M., Stetson, S. J., Jimenez, S., Entman, M. L., Noon, G. P., Bowles, N. E., Towbin, J. A., and Torre-Amione, G. 3-3-2004 Molecular normalization of dystrophin in the failing left and right ventricle of patients treated with either pulsatile or continuous flow-type ventricular assist devices J.Am.Coll.Cardiol. 43:(5) 811-817

Weber, C. R., Piacentino, V., III, Ginsburg, K. S., Houser, S. R., and Bers, D. M. 8-2-2002 Na(+)-Ca(2+) exchange current and submembrane [Ca(2+)] during the cardiac action potential Circ.Res. 90:(2) 182-189

Welch, S., Plank, D., Witt, S., Glascock, B., Schaefer, E., Chimenti, S., Andreoli, A. M., Limana, F., Leri, A., Kajstura, J., Anversa, P., and Sussman, M. A. 5-4-2002 Cardiac-specific IGF-1 expression attenuates dilated cardiomyopathy in tropomodulin-overexpressing transgenic mice Circ.Res. 90:(6) 641-648

Wickenden, A. D., Kaprielian, R., Kassiri, Z., Tsoporis, J. N., Tsushima, R., Fishman, G. I., and Backx, P. H. 1998 The role of action potential prolongation and altered intracellular calcium handling in the pathogenesis of heart failure Cardiovasc.Res. 37:(2) 312-323

Wilson, E. M. and Spinale, F. G. 2001 Myocardial remodelling and matrix metalloproteinases in heart failure: turmoil within the interstitium Ann.Med. 33:(9) 623-634

Wohlschlaeger, J., Levkau, B., Brockhoff, G., Schmitz, K. J., von, Winterfeld M., Takeda, A., Takeda, N., Stypmann, J., Vahlhaus, C., Schmid, C., Pomjanski, N., Bocking, A., and Baba, H. A. 2-3-2010 Hemodynamic support by left ventricular assist devices reduces cardiomyocyte DNA content in the failing human heart Circulation 121:(8) 989-996

Wohlschlaeger, J., von, Winterfeld M., Milting, H., El, Banayosy A., Schmitz, K. J., Takeda, A., Takeda, N., Azhari, P., Schmid, C., August, C., Schmid, K. W., and Baba, H. A. 2008 Decreased myocardial chromogranin a expression and colocalization with brain natriuretic peptide during reverse cardiac remodeling after ventricular unloading J.Heart Lung Transplant. 27:(4) 442-449

Woodiwiss, A. J., Tsotetsi, O. J., Sprott, S., Lancaster, E. J., Mela, T., Chung, E. S., Meyer, T. E., and Norton, G. R. 2-1-2001 Reduction in myocardial collagen cross-linking parallels left ventricular dilatation in rat models of systolic chamber dysfunction Circulation 103:(1) 155-160

Xydas, S., Kherani, A. R., Chang, J. S., Klotz, S., Hay, I., Mutrie, C. J., Moss, G. W., Gu, A., Schulman, A. R., Gao, D., Hu, D., Wu, E. X., Wei, C., Oz, M. C., and Wang, J. 2006 beta(2)-Adrenergic stimulation attenuates left ventricular remodeling, decreases apoptosis, and improves calcium homeostasis in a rodent model of ischemic cardiomyopathy J Pharmacol.Exp Ther. 317:(2) 553-561

Yancy, C. W., Fowler, M. B., Colucci, W. S., Gilbert, E. M., Bristow, M. R., Cohn, J. N., Lukas, M. A., Young, S. T., and Packer, M. 3-5-2001 Race and the response to adrenergic blockade with carvedilol in patients with chronic heart failure N.Engl.J.Med. 344:(18) 1358-1365

Young, J. B. 2001 Healing the heart with ventricular assist device therapy: mechanisms of cardiac recovery Ann.Thorac.Surg. 71:(3 Suppl) S210-S219

Zafeiridis, A., Jeevanandam, V., Houser, S. R., and Margulies, K. B. 18-8-1998 Regression of cellular hypertrophy after left ventricular assist device support 22 Circulation 98:(7) 656-662

Zhang, Q., Xiang, J., Wang, X., Liu, H., Hu, B., Feng, M., and Fu, Q. 2010 Beta(2)-adrenoceptor agonist clenbuterol reduces infarct size and myocardial apoptosis after myocardial ischaemia/reperfusion in anaesthetized rats Br.J.Pharmacol. 160:(6) 1561-1572

6

Risk Factor Analysis and Management of Cerebrovascular Accidents in Japanese Patients Supported by Left Ventricular Assist Device

Tomoko S. Kato, Kazuo Komamura, Ikutaro Nakajima,
Ayako Takahashi, Noboru Oda and Masafumi Kitakaze
National Cerebral and Cardiovascular Center
Japan

1. Introduction

Heart transplantation provides considerable survival benefits for patients with end-stage heart failure, but it is available for only a small fraction of these patients due to donor shortage. Especially in Japan, domestic legal issues had severely limited the number of heart transplantation until the Revised Organ Transplant Law was launched in 2010. The mean waiting period of Japanese heart transplant candidates after left ventricular assist device (LVAD) surgery had exceeded 2 years and occasionally reached 4 years until recently (Sasaoka T et al., 2010).

The long-term LVAD support can result in serious complications such as cerebrovascular accident (CVA), the most common cause of death following LVAD surgery (Rose EA et al., 2001; Holman WL, 2009; Saito S, et al. 2010). CVA is the leading cause of death and the primary reason for elimination from transplant eligibility. In addition, transplant recipients with a history of CVA face tremendous difficulties in being reintegrated into society, often for years after transplant (Nakajima I et al., 2011).

Therefore, we investigated factors associated with CVA after LVAD surgery in Japanese patients, as well as we reviewed our treatment strategies for CVA and the outcome of these patients after developing CVA.

2. Special circumstance surrounding transplant and LVAD issues in Japan

Until recently, brain-death tests, conducted on the premise of organ donation, were only for possible donors aged over 15 with formally signed donor cards indicating a willingness to donate his or her organs. The cardiac donation rate per million population in Japan is only 0.08 or less than 10 cases in the nation, whereas it is 7.3 in the United States, 5.3 in Spain, and 0.97 in South Korea in 2007 (Fukushima N et al., 2009; Hashimoto S et al., 2011).

Furthermore, only one pulsatile extracorporeal left ventricular assist device (LVAD) (Toyobo-LVAS®, Nipro Corp., Tokyo, Japan, Figure 1) was covered by the National Health

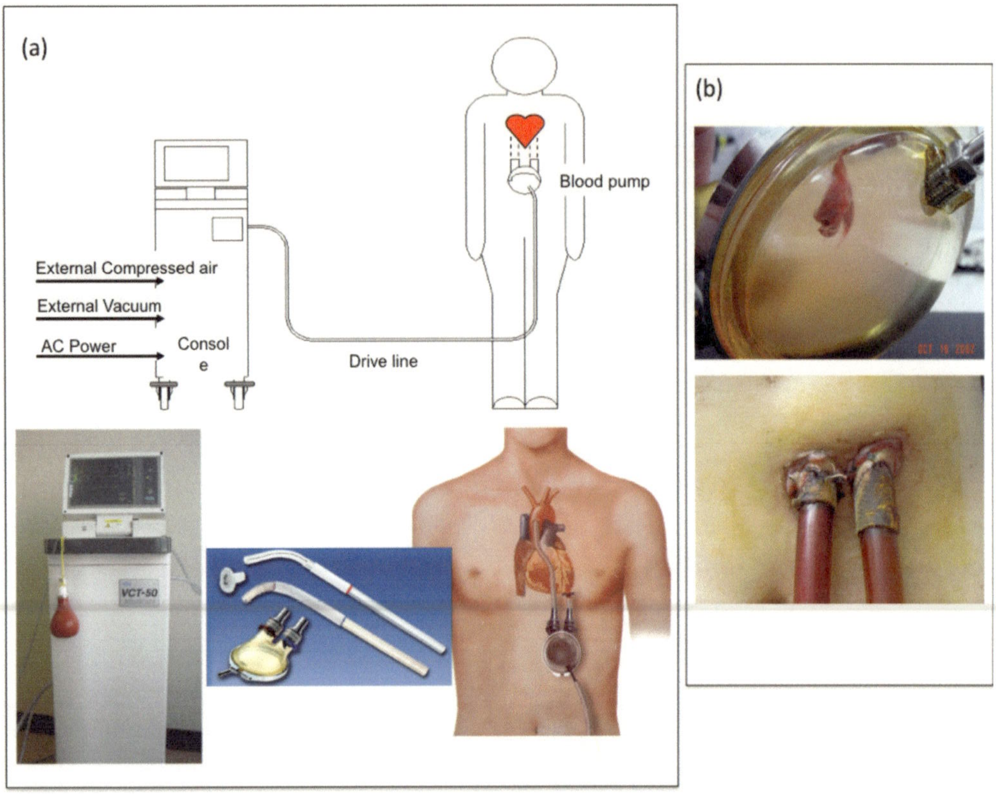

Fig. 1. (a) Outline of the Toyobo-LVAS® system with device console (left lower panel), blood pumps and inflow/outflow cannula (middle lower panel) and the chart of the LVAD system (right lower panel). The blood pump consisted of a diaphragm with a pulsatile flow through two mechanical valves, operated by a pneumatically driven system. The maximum stroke volume was 70 mL per beat when testing with water. The blood contacting surface is covered by segmented polyurethane approved for medical use. (b) Representative pictures of the blood pump with mobile thrombi (upper panel) and a granulating wound at the penetration sites of the inflow/outflow cannula in the abdominal skin

Insurance System as of November 2010 (Sasaoka T et al., 2010). Some implantable LVAD were used for Japanese patients for the purpose of clinical trail, or when medical expense was paid individually. Therefore, as improbable as it may sound, Japanese patients with advanced heart failure were being maintained mainly by pulsatile extracorporeal Toyobo-LVAS® as a "bridge-to-transplant" treatment for 2 to 4 years until being transplanted. Needless to say, some of them died while on the device. Given these circumstances, our long-term management skills for overcoming LVAD-related complications have improved over time, with the 1-year survival now being 82% (Sasaoka T et al., 2010). However, even with this success rate of survival, CVA still remains the leading cause of death.

The Toyobo-LVAS® was actually designed for "short-term" support, but the lack of alternatives resulted in it becoming a "long-term" support device in Japan. The Toyobo-LVAS® also requires an intensive anti-coagulation therapy, such as a target prothrombin time-international normalized ratio of 3.0-4.0. The 3-month and 1-year CVA-free survival rate for a patient with Toyobo-LVAS® is 56.1% and 36.8%, respectively (Sasaoka T et al.,

2010; Nakajima et al., 2011). The overall incidence of CVA for Toyobo-LVAS® patients was reported as 57.3 % at a mean observation period of 224 days, and a report from another institution indicated a CVA incidence of 53.6% at a mean of 505 days (Nakajima et al., 2011; Saito et al., 2009).

In spite of such a high frequency of CVA development after Toyobo-LVAS® surgery, we could achieve a reasonably high survival rate after the device placement thanks to the use of prothrombin complex concentrate (PCC) for rapid reversal of warfarin-induced anticoagulation in this population (Takahashi A et al., 2010). We here describe (i) factors associated with CVA after LVAD surgery in Japanese patients in order to distinguish patients with high risks for CVA, and (ii) the effects of PCC for rapid reversal of warfarin-induced anticoagulation in patients developing hemorrhagic stroke who were supported by LVAD, based on our experience.

3. Pre- and post-operative risk factors associated with CVA developments in Japanese patients supported by left ventricular assist device

3.1 Risk factors for CVA at any time after LVAD surgery

Nakajima et al. reviewed a total of 118 adult Japanese patients who were supported by LVAD between 1994 and 2009 (Nakajima et al., 2011). A CVA was defined as an ischemic or hemorrhagic intracranial event that persisted beyond 24 hours or less than 24 hours with infarction on an image study, based on the Interagency Registry for Mechanically Assisted Circulatory Support (INTERMACS) adverse events definitions of stroke. Clinical characteristics, hemodynamic data, and laboratory indexes associated with CVA after LVAD surgery were analyzed.

In total, 57 (48.3%) patients developed CVA 133.5±184.7 days after surgery. Patients who developed CVA revealed to have longer duration of heart failure ($p=0.0039$), more frequency of cardiomyopathy as a baseline heart disease vs myocarditis/acute coronary syndrome ($p=0.039$), more frequency of undergoing surgery with inflow cannula site at the left atrium ($p=0.011$), and longer duration of inotropic requirement after surgery ($p<0.0001$) than those who did not develop CVA. In addition, patients with CVA had higher pre-LVAD mean right atrial pressure (mRA) ($p=0.001$), higher pre-LVAD total bilirubin (T-Bil) concentration ($p=0.024$), lower lymphocyte subset percentage ($p=0.019$), lower pre-LVAD total protein (TP) concentration ($p=0.001$) and larger pre-LVAD right ventricular end-diastolic dimension (RVEDD) on echocardiogram ($p=0.0003$). This combination could discriminate patients developing CVA from those not developing CVA at any time after surgery with a predictive accuracy of 71.8%, which the following formula;

$$z=-0.507566 + (1.5664\times \text{[baseline heart disease; 1=cardiomyopathy, 0=other diseases]}) + (3.49143\times \text{[type of LVAD; 1=left atrium drainage Toyobo®, 0=other type of LVAD]} + (0.123626\times mRA) + (0.185355\times T\text{-}Bil) - (1.04891\times TP) + (0.153542\times RVEDD).$$

where $Z > 0$ indicates patients developing CVA and $Z < 0$ indicates patients not developing CVA after LVAD surgery.

The above finding could be implicated that patients with longstanding heart failure associated with malnutrition as well as accompanied right heart failure would be at higher risk for CVA development after LVAD surgery.

Hierarchical multiple regression analysis for the interactions between CVA associated factors revealed that duration of heart failure and pre-LVAD lymphocyte subset influenced the duration of inotropic support after surgery, which in turn influenced CVA development.

Accordingly, both duration of heart failure and lymphocyte subset before surgery were indirectly associated with CVA. In addition, right ventricular size had an effect on the duration of inotropic support in addition to its direct effect on CVA development (Figure 2a).

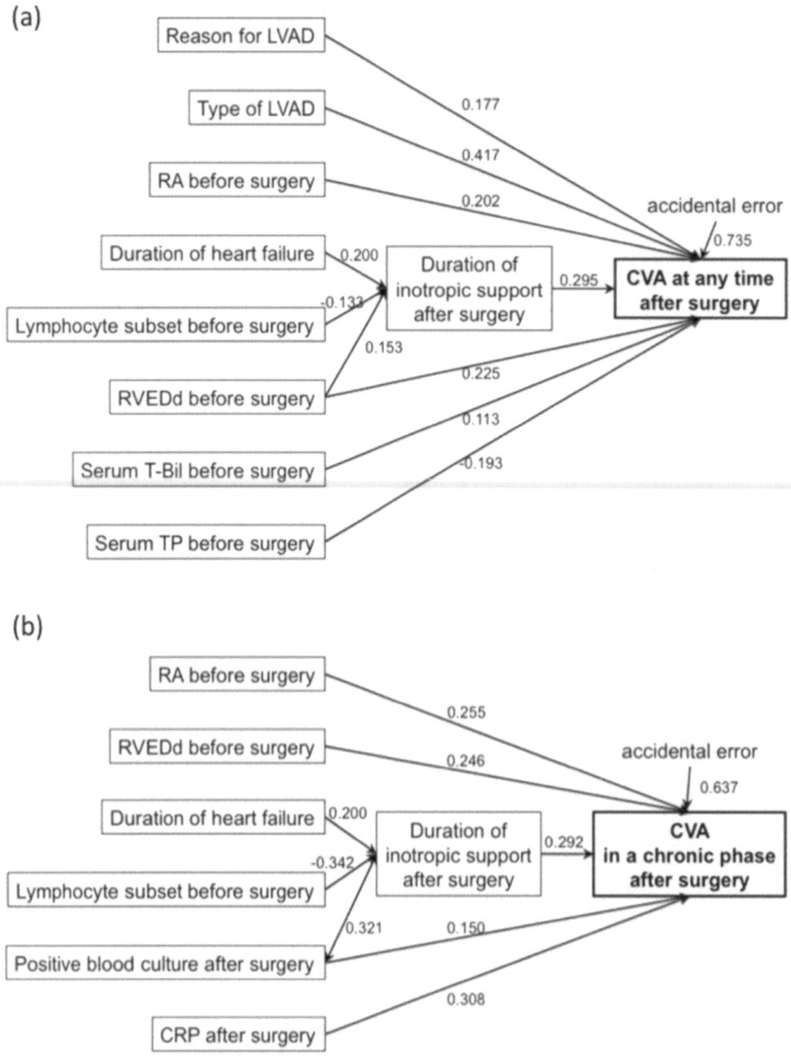

Fig. 2. (a) A path diagram based on the hierarchical multiple regression analysis for all studied patients. Observed variables are delineated by squares. Unidirectional arrows indicate cause-and-effect relationships. The number next to each arrow indicates the path coefficient of the standard partial regression coefficient. The regression error is added without delineation. (b)The path diagram based on the hierarchical multiple regression analysis for patients survived longer than 3 months without CVA. Observed variables are delineated by squares. Unidirectional arrows indicate cause-and-effect relationships. Bidirectional arrows indicate reciprocal cause-and-effect relationships. The number next to each arrow indicates the path coefficient of the standard partial regression coefficient. The regression error is added without delineation. (Adopted from Nakajima et al. Circ J)

3.2 Risk factors for CVA in a chronic phase after LVAD surgery

Because of the long waiting period supported by LVAD for transplant such as beyond 2 years in Japan, a certain amount of patients develop CVA in a chronic phase after LVAD surgery. Therefore, Nakajima et al. also performed the analysis to find factors associated with CVA in the chronic phase after surgery by excluding patients who had CVA in an acute phase or who had died within 3 months after surgery.

For this sub-analysis, duration of heart failure was longer ($p=0.012$), myocardial fibrosis was severer ($p=0.034$), duration of post-LVAD inotropic requirement was longer ($p<0.0001$), mRA was higher ($p=0.0005$), the pre-LVAD lymphocyte subset of peripheral blood was lower ($p=0.008$), and pre-LVAD RVEDD was larger ($p=0.0006$) in patients with CVA later than 3 months from the surgery compared to those who never developed CVA after surgery. In addition, the proportion of patients who had positive blood cultures was higher ($p=0.0002$) in patients who developed CVA in a chronic phase. The post-LVAD serum creatinine concentration ($p=0.011$) and C-reactive protein level (CRP) ($p<0.0001$) were higher in patients who developed CVA in a chronic phase than who never developed CVA after surgery.

A discriminant function test revealed that a discriminant score (Z) defined using the following equation yielded the discriminant probability of 85.9 %:

$$z=-10.0754 + (0.212146\times \text{mRA}) + (0.179936\times \text{RVEDd}) + (2.03552\times [\text{blood culture positivity after surgery; 1=positive, 0=negative}]) + (0.787837\times \text{CRP})$$

where $Z > 0$ indicates 3 months survivors after LVAD surgery developing CVA subsequently and $Z < 0$ indicates patients would never develop CVA.

The hierarchical analysis for evaluating interactions of factors associated with chronic phase CVA again revealed that both duration of heart failure and lymphocyte subset before surgery were indirectly associated with CVA through their effect on duration of inotropic support after surgery (Figure 2b). Here again, patients with longstanding heart failure associated with accompanied right heart failure and those with post-operative infection would be at higher risk for developing CVA in a chronic phase after LVAD surgery.

Multivariate regression analysis for CVA at any time after surgery and CVA in a chronic phase after surgery were shown in Table 1.

Although the population of the above study was different from heart failure patients in the US or European countries, the combination of pre-LVAD right heart failure and post-LVAD infection contribute to chronic phase CVA after surgery is worthwhile information.

4. Prothrombin complex concentrate for rapid reversal of warfarin-induced anticoagulation in patients with hemorrhagic stroke supported by left ventricular assist device

4.1 Prothrombin complex concentrate

Development of hemorrhagic stroke is one of the most serious complications in patients supported by LVAD, who require extensive oral anticoagulant therapy (Leitz K et al. , 2007). Hemorrhagic stroke associated with anticoagulation has a high mortality, and more than 50% of patients die within 30 days (Sjöblom L et al., 2001). Thus, warfarin-related hemorrhagic stroke is considered a medical emergency especially for patients supported by LVAD. Nevertheless, there are no guidelines for reversal of anticoagulation for such patients.

Parameter	OR (95% CI)	Discriminant score (95% CI)	*p* value
Associated factors for overall CVA development at any time after surgery			
cardiomyopathy	4.79 (1.31-17.4)	1.56 (0.28-2.86)	0.018
left atrium drainage Toyobo®	32.8 (8.39-128.4)	3.49 (2.12-4.86)	<0.0001
Mean RA before surgery (mmHg)	1.13 (1.04-1.23)	0.12 (0.04-0.21)	0.005
T-Bil before surgery (mg/dL)	1.20 (0.95-1.52)	0.18 (-0.05-0.41)	0.12
TP before surgery (mg/dL)	0.35 (0.17-0.74)	-1.05 [-1.80-(-0.30)]	0.006
RVEDd before surgery (mm)	1.17 (1.07-1.28)	0.15(0.06-0.24)	0.001
Associated factors for chronic phase CVA development			
Mean RA before surgery (mmHg)	1.24 (1. 07-1.42)	0.21 (0.07-0.35)	0.004
RVEDd before surgery (mm)	1.20 (1.06-1.34)	0.18 (0.05-0.31)	0.006
blood culture positive after surgery	7.66 (1.50-39.0)	2.04 (0.41-3.66)	0.015
CRP after surgery (mg/dL)	2.19 (1.47-3.25)	0.78 (0.39-1.18)	0.0002

Table 1. Multivariate stepwise forward selection analysis of associated factors for CVA. (Adopted from Nakajima et al. Circ J 2011)

The anticoagulation effect of warfarin is related to its ability to inhibit synthesis of the vitamin K-dependent clotting factors II, VII, IX, and X. The appropriate way to reverse the anticoagulation effect of warfarin depends on the clinical situation. Minor or asymptomatic bleeding needs a less aggressive reversal, whereas serious bleeding requires rapid reversal to avoid succeeding fatal events, regardless of the reason for anticoagulation. For major bleeding, guidelines recommend the administration of vitamin K (5 mg i.v. or oral), and/or PCC (50 U/kg), and/or FFP (15 ml/kg) (British Committee for Standards in Haematology. 1998; Ansell J et al., 2001).

However, reversing warfarin-induced anticoagulation by vitamin K is time consuming (Aguilar MI et al., 2007). Reversing anticoagulation with vitamin K requires 4 to 24 hours, then might cause a fatal situation after hemorrhagic events, and also its persistent effect may promote clot formation. Thus, vitamin K administration is not an adequate treatment as an emergent treatment to stop further bleeding for patients with intracranial haemorrhages supported by LVAD.

The administration of fresh frozen plasma (FFP) requires substantial intravenous volume (Aguilar MI et al., 2007), which is not adequate for patients with heart failure. Prothrombin complex concentrate (PCC), which contains a high concentration of the vitamin K-dependent coagulation factors II, VII, IX, and X, has been reported to be effective for rapid reversal of warfarin-induced anticoagulation. The PCC promotes a much more rapid reversal of (PT)- international normalized ratio (INR) than FFP or/and vitamin K (Steiner T et al., 2006; Aguilar MI et al., 2007) which is explained by its higher concentration of coagulation factors than FFP. The PCC product (PPSB-HT®; Nihon Pharmaceuticals, Tokyo, Japan) became available at our institution since 2001, and it has been used for emergency reversal of warfarin-induced anticoagulation such as hemorrhagic stroke, intraabdominal haemorrhage and cardiac tamponade.

4.2 Our experience of using prothrombin complex concentrate

Takahashi et al. reviewed 38 consecutive hemorrhagic stroke events occurred in patients supported by LVAD for bridge-to-transplantation between 1996 and 2007 at National Cerebrovascular Center, Osaka, Japan (Takahashi A et al., 2010). Fourteen hemorrhagic strokes were treated by FFP and 24 hemorrhagic strokes were treated by PCC. The FFP was initially administrated after the evens at the dosage of body weight (kg) × 0.08 × (100-hematocrit/100) × 0.3 × 0.2 × 1000 (ml). If the PT-INR was still greater than 2 after the initial FFP administration, additional FFP was administrated. In patients who were treated with PCC, the initial dosage of 500 to 1000 units were administered for 30 to 60 minutes, and if the INR was greater than 2 after the initial PCC administration, additional PCC was administrated. The proportion of patients' survival after the hemorrhagic stroke was significantly smaller in those treated with FFP administration than those who were treated with PCC (35.7% vs. 75.0%, $p < 0.05$). Only 18% of patients who were treated with FFP could be back on the transplant waiting list, while 58% of patients treated with PCC could be back on the waiting list. None of the patients who were only treated with FFP and not received PCC were able to undergo heart transplantation, whereas 21.4% patients who were treated with PCC successfully underwent heart transplantation.

Representative computed tomography scans from a patient treated with FFP and a patients receiving PCC were shown in Figure 3.

Several studies demonstrated the effect of recombinant activated factor VII on warfarin reversal and reported successful results treating hemorrhagic stroke events (Deveras RAE et al., 2002). Further studies are required to establish the difference of the effect of warfarin reversal between PCCs and recombinant activated factor VII.

5. Conclusion

Patients' general condition including malnutrition, in addition to device selection, would contribute to overall CVA development after surgery. In the chronic phase after surgery, pre-LVAD right heart failure and post-LVAD systemic infection were highly associated with CVA development. It was noteworthy that post-operative infection was selected as discriminating factors for CVA development in a chronic phase. An association of right heart dysfunction with a high mortality rate after LVAD surgery has been reported, although the association between pre-LVAD right heart failure and post-LVAD CVA was not fully evaluated. The longstanding heart failure might cause not only biventricular failure but also systemic vascular dysfunction including cerebral blood vessel. In addition, patients with biventricular failure required a long duration of inotropic support after LVAD. Long-term inotropic dependency due to right heart failure might cause line infections leading to systemic infection.

This unique situation surrounding LVAD issues in Japan may have influenced the results of this study, especially with respect to early postoperative outcome. The number of patients on devices as a 'destination therapy' has been increasing worldwide. Even in the era of new generation devices, CVA remains to be important complication. In that sense, we believe that the information described in this chapter are helpful in the long-term management strategies from the perspective of CVA risk stratification in patients on destination therapy devices.

Administration of PCC can result in a prompt reversal of warfarin-induced anticoagulation, and could be of importance for the survival of patients supported by LVAD, who require intensified anticoagulation therapy and who are at high risk for hemorrhagic stroke.

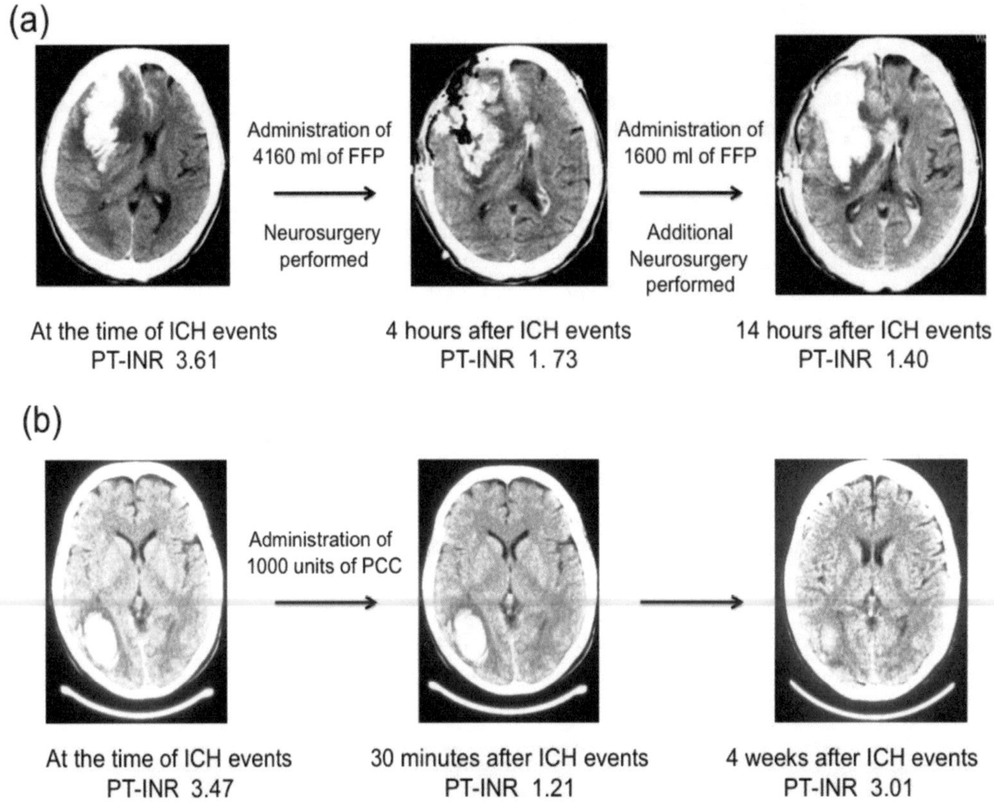

Fig. 3. Representative images of computed tomography head scan from patients in Group FFP (a) and in Group PCC (b). (a) A 50-year-old male developed ICH in the right frontal lobe with a PT-INR of 3.61. After 4160 ml of FFP administration resulting in PT-INR of 1.73, the patients required neurosurgery. Due to residual ICH, the patient required additional neurosurgery but eventually died. (b) A 41-year-old female developed ICH in the right posterior lobe with a PT-INR of 3.47. The immediate administration of 1000 units of PCC resulted in the PT-INR of 1.21 within 20 minutes. The patient underwent heart transplantation 2.8 years after the ICH event without neurological after-effects

6. Acknowledgement

The year 2010 was the dawn of a new era of LVAD/transplant issues in Japan. In December 2010, implantable continuous-flow LVADs [Evaheart™ (Sun Medical Corp, Nagano, Japan) and DuraHeart™ (Terumo Heart Inc, Tokyo, Japan)] finally obtained Manufacture and Sales approval from the Ministry of Health, Labor, and Welfare. The Revised Organ Transplant Law went into effect in July 2010, allowing both adults and children to have a chance to be donors as well as recipients. The number of transplants has dramatically increased since then. Until the revision of the Organ Transplant Law, a number of Japanese patients chose to undergo transplantation abroad, mostly in the US or Europe. We all Japanese would like to express our deep appreciation to the entire European/US populations for accepting Japanese patients as their transplant recipients to date.

7. References

Aguilar MI, Hart RG, Kase CS, et al. Treatment of warfarin-associated intracerebral haemorrhage: literature review and expert opinion. Mayo Clin Proc 2007; 82:82–92.

Ansell J, Hirsh J, Dalen J, Bussey H, et al. Managing Oral Anticoagulant Therapy. Chest 2001; 119:22S–38S

British Committee for Standards in Haematology. Guidelines on oral anticoagulation: third edition. Br J Haematol 1998; 101:374–87.

Deveras RAE, Kessler CM. Reversal of Warfarin-Induced Excessive Anticoagulation with Recombinant Human Factor VIIa Concentrate. Ann Intern Med. 2002. 137: 884-888.

Fukushima N, Ono M, Nakatani T, Minami M, Konaka S, Ashikari J. Strategies for maximizing heart and lung transplantation opportunities in Japan. Transplant Proc. 2009; 41: 273-6.

Hashimoto S, Kato TS, Komamura K, Hanatani A, Niwaya K, Funatsu T, Nakatani T, Kobayashi J, Sumita Y, Tanaka N, Hashimura K, Asakura M, Kanzaki H, Kitakaze M. J Cardiology. 2011 Jan; 57:215-22.

Holman WL, Kormos RL, Naftel DC, Miller MA, Pagani FD, Blume E, Cleeton T, Koenig SC, Edwards L, Kirklin JK. Predictors of death and transplant in patients with a mechanical circulatory support device: a multi-institutional study. J Heart Lung Transplant 2009; 28:44-50.

Lietz K, Long JW, Kfoury AG, et al. Outcome of LVAS as Destination Therapy. Outcomes of left ventricular assist device implantation as destination therapy in the post-REMATCH era: implications for patient selection. Circulation 2007; 116:497–505.

Nakajima I, Kato TS, Komamura K, Takahashi A, Oda N, Sasaoka T, Asakura M, Hashimura K, Kitakaze M. Pre- and Post-Operative Risk Factors Associated With Cerebrovascular Accidents in Patients Supported by Left Ventricular Assist Device. Circ J 2011; 75: 1138 - 1146.

Oda N, Kato TS, Komamura K, Hanatani A, Mano A, Hashimura K, Asakura M, Niwaya K, Funatsu T, Kobayashi J, Wada K, Hashimoto S, Ishibashi-Ueda H, Nakano Y, Kihara Y, Kitakaze M. Clinical course and outcome of heart transplant recipients: single center experience at the National Cardiovascular Center in Japan. Int Heart J. 2010; 51:264-71.

Oda N, Kato TS, Komamura K, Patel J, Kobashigawa JA. Retrospective review of Japanese patients undergoing heart transplantation in Japan compared with those undergoing transplantation in the United States. J Heart Lung Transplant. 2010; 29:1076-8.

Rose EA, Gelijns AC, Moskowitz AJ, Heitjan DF, Stevenson LW, Dembitsky W, et al.; Randomized Evaluation of Mechanical Assistance for the Treatment of Congestive Heart Failure (REMATCH) Study Group. Long-term mechanical left ventricular assistance for end-stage heart failure. N Engl J Med 2001; 15; 345:1435-43.

Saito S, Matsumiya G, Sakaguchi T, Miyagawa S, Yoshikawa Y, Yamauchi T, Kuratani T, Sawa Y. Risk factor analysis of long-term support with left ventricular assist system. Circ J. 2010 25; 74:715-22.

Saito S, Matsumiya G, Sakaguchi T, Fujita T, Kuratani T, Ichikawa H, et al. Fifteen-year experience with Toyobo paracorporeal left ventricular assist system. J Artif Organs. 2009; 12:27-34.

Sasaoka T, Kato TS (corresponding), Komamura K, Takahashi A, Nakajima I, Oda N, Hanatani A, Mano A, Asakura M, Hashimura K, Niwaya K, Funatsu T, Kobayashi J, Kitamura S, Shishido T, Wada K, Miyata S, Nakatani T, Isobe M, Kitakaze M. Improved Long-Term Performance of Pulsatile Extracorporeal Left Ventricular Assist Device. J Cardiology 2010; 56: 220-228.

Sjöblom L, Hårdemark HG, Lindgren A, et al. Management and prognostic features of intracerebral haemorrhage during anticoagulant therapy: a Swedish multicenter study. Stroke 2001; 32:2567–74.

Steiner T, Rosand J, Diringer M. Intracerebral haemorrhage associated with oral anticoagulant therapy: current practices and unresolved questions. Stroke 2006; 37:256–62.

Takahashi A, Kato TS, Oda N, Komamura K, Kanzaki H, Asakura M, Hashimura K, Niwaya K, Funatsu T, Nakatani T, Kobaashi J, Kitamura S, Shishido T, Miyata S, Takahashi J, Iihara K, Kitakaze M. Prothrombin Complex Concentrate for Rapid Reversal of Warfarin-Induced Anticoagulation in Patients with Intracerebral Haemorrhages Supported by Left Ventricular Assist Device. International Journal of Gerontology 2010; 4: 143–147.

7

Ventricular Assist Devices for Pediatric Heart Disease

Cenk Eray Yildiz
*Istanbul University, Institute of Cardiology,
Department of Cardiovascular Surgery, Istanbul,
Turkey*

1. Introduction

Mechanical Circulation Assist Devices are designed for the treatment of acute and chronic heart failure and can be applied for different indications and assist period. Treatments that are carried out with Ventricular Assist Device System (VADs) have improved over course of time, within the practical applications of pediatric cardiac surgery. Pulsatile devices being in the lead, paracorporeal assist devices and implantable ventricular assist devices all have fields of application. However, ECMO (Extracorporeal Membrane Oxygenator) treatment is still applied on infants and children. These systems are preferred to assist patients with respiratory failure after heart surgery. But, this assist remains for a short term and compulsorily puts the patients into intensive care. In recent years, so many new devices have been developed, such as easily intubated cannulas for children including infants and miniature pumps for pediatric use. These devices are recommended for mid and long term, which is more predominant than ECMO. They are applied successfully to assist bridge to recovery and bridge to transplantation. Here, an assessment is made for different types of contemporary devices, decision making and application strategy, device technology, implantation techniques, anticoagulation and follow-up, new generation assist devices that operate with pediatric ventricular assist device for the treatment of pediatric heart failure. Proverbially, in spite of the successful results, ECMO and centrifugal pumps are not suitable for every patient because of the reasons such as long period of stays in intensive care unit, lack of mobilization and shortness of operating time. VAD systems are developed for little children of previously which only ECMO was suitable for. With the VAD treatment of selected pediatric population, especially in the cases of myocarditis and cardiomyopathy, mobilization and low anticoagulation have been enabled and resulted in 90 % of survival rate. VAD is preferred instead of ECMO and if there is a need for circulation assist that exceeds 1-2 weeks, the complication rate decreases. These devices get more reliable day by day and they will play an effective role in future as a treatment method for the complex congenital heart diseases that aim for transplantation or bridging treatment for cardiac recuperation. Eventually, what is dreamt for future is to attain permanent solutions.

2. History of mechanical support device in pediatrics

In 1974 Bartlett reported the use of extracorporeal membrane oxygenation in pediatric patients with respiratory failure or after repair of congenital heart disease. Bartlett first used the ECMO device on a neonate and named it "Esperanza", meaning "Hope" (Bartlett et al., 1977). In 1980 Pollock reported the first use of an intraaortic balloon pump in children (Pollock et al., 1980). In 1983, Veasy reported the use of small balloon catheters in 15 children (Veasy et al., 1983). The Thoratec ventricular assist devices have been available since the early 1980s, and can be implanted in children and adolescents (Reinhartz et al, 2001). The first neonatal oxygenator was released in the 1990s (Duncan, 2001).

In spite of the success of ventricular assist devices for adults, not much has been done to develop similar devices for pediatric population. Afterwards, in 1992, the "Berlin Heart" offered the first commercially available system with miniaturized paracorporeal pumps and cannulae. The first implantation of a Medos ventricular assist device as a bridging to transplantation took place in 1994 (Konertz, 2001). The DeBakey VAD Child (MicroMed Technology, Inc. Houston, TX) became available for use in 2004 (Morales et al., 2005).

In 1989, it was reported by ELSO (Extracorporeal Life Support Organization) that the number of centers that use ECMO was 100 worldwide. Until 2005, more than 30.000 patients, with the support of ECMO, have survived with 65 % success rate (ECLS Registry, 2005). ECLS registry in 2008 provides a database of 37.000 patients from all around the world with details about demographic factors, diagnosis, treatment and complications (Haines et al., 2009). There have been studies with 80 % success for the usage of ECMO on infants with acute hypoxemic respiratory failure (Field et al., 1996). On infants that undergo traditional treatments, the survival rate is 30 %. With ECMO support, this rate is doubled (Bennett et al., 2001). Currently, the support devices are applied on infants and children with uncontrollable heart failure. Final ECLS, ECMO guideline has been published in April 2009. In this chapter, we will be discussing ECMO as a cardiac support device and as well as other mechanical cardiac support devices applied on child patients.

3. The selection of mechanical support devices

The selection of suitable mechanical support device is determined according to the surface area of the body. Mechanical support indication depends on the predetermining the length of time between bridging treatment and transplantation, effect of the disease, pathophysiological events and the fact that many organizations can obtain different devices. Although there have been a variety of cardiac support systems for adult patients, the devices for neonates and infants are scarce. Today, two of the the most common methods for the short term cardiac support for infants are ECMO and Centrifugal Extracorporeal VAD (Ventricular Assist Device) (Table 1). Nowadays, the presence of new paracorporeal VAD is encouraging. The technical specifications of mechanical cardiac devices used for children are summarized in Table 2. These systems are used in bridging treatment that extends the transplantation period a few months. Since the case is completed, intra-aortic balloon pump (IABP) will be discussed, although it is rare for pediatric patients.

3.1 Extracorporeal membrane oxygenation (ECMO)

ECMO is the most important assist system for mechanical heart support for pediatric population. There are two major methods: veno-venous ECMO, which provides ventilator

	ECMO	VAD
Oxygenator	Yes	No
Circulation	Long, with reservoir	Short, no reservoir
Anticoagulation	ACT 180-220 seconds	ACT 140-160 seconds
Air emboli	Low	High (L-VDC)
Support type	Cardiorespiratory	Cardiac
Ventricular decompression	Atrial septestomy/LA vent	Not required
Length of Support	A few weeks	Weeks
Cannulation	Transthoracic or jugular	Transthoracic

Table 1. Comparison of ECMO and centrifugal extracorporeal VAD

Device type	Intra-aortic baloon pump	ECMO	Centri-fugal pump	Berlin Heart Excor	Medos HIA VAD	Thoratec II	HeartMate IP/VE	Abiomed BVS 5000
Position	Intraaortic	External	External	External	External	External	External	External
Ventri-cular support	Left	Double	Left, right or double	Left, right or double	Left, right or double	Left, right or double	Left	Left, right or double
Duration	Short	Short	Short	Long	Short	Medium Long	Long	Medium
Flow	Pulsatile	Non - pulsatile	Non - pulsatile	Pulsatile	Pulsatile	Pulsatile	Pulsatile	Pulsatile
Power Supply	Pneumatic	Electrical	Electrical	Pneumatic	Pneumatic	Pneumatic	Electrical or Pneumatic	Pneumatic
Cannu-lation	Peripheric Artery	Peripheric Artery and Ven	Central or Peri-pheric	Central	Central	Central or Peripheric	Central	Central
Anticoa-gulation	Not required	Required	Not required or low	Required	Required	Required	Not required	Required
Mobili-zation	No	No	No	Yes	No	Yes, limited	No	No
Discharge from hospital	No	No	No	No	No	Yes	Yes	No

Table 2. Technical specification of mechanical cardiac assist devices for pediatric patients

support and the other one is veno-arterial ECMO, which is suitable for patients with circulatory failure and it provides both heart and lung support. ECMO is more advantageous than other devices in terms of its usage for patients with bi-ventricular failure, respiratory insufficiency and pulmonary hypertension. Discharge survival rate of a short term ECMO treated patient is 40-80% (Bartlett et al., 1977). If the recovery time is prolonged, risk of infection increases. Since there is a complication incidence, the usage of ECMO is limited within a few feeks (max. 4-6 weeks) (Cahturvedi et al., 2004). For the patients that require a longer assistance, other types of ventricular assist devices may be suitable.

Reports of a center's experience usually find that conditions of complex heart disease with either excess pulmonary blood flow or decreased pulmonary blood flow constitute the majority of cases requiring ECMO for pediatric cardiac support (Duncan et al., 1999). The most common scenarios for support usually occur in children after cardiac surgery, namely, failure to wean from cardiopulmonary bypass and cardiogenic shock or cardiac arrest occurring in the intensive care unit postoperatively (Delius et al., 1992; Hunkeler et al., 1992; Raithel et al., 1992). However, nonresponsive medical conditions also occur in children that require mechanical circulatory support (Duncan et al., 2001; Del Nido et al., 1994). Conditions that represent contraindications for ECMO are now often successfully supported. For instance, patients with shunted single ventricle physiology, were often denied ECMO in the past due to difficulties in achieving balance between the pulmonary and systemic circulations. Due to improvements, ECMO and VADs are currently necessary adjuncts for the successful surgical approach to these patients (Darling et al., 2001; Pizarro et al., 2001).

Since its launch, ECMO has been the predominant form of support for children. Due to the presence of an oxygenator in the circuit, ECMO is most useful in providing support when heart disease is accompanied by hypoxia and pulmonary hypertension. The presence of an oxygenator and other complexities of the ECMO circuit require higher levels of anticoagulation (Hetzer et al., 1998).

Another important difference between devices is the impact on recovery of ventricular function during support. Experimental studies have shown increased ventricular wall stress during ECMO support while VADs provide better ventricular unloading leading to decreased wall stress (Ratcliffe et al., 1991). ECMO may also contribute to ongoing myocardial damage during support by providing desaturated blood flow to the coronary arteries (Kato et al., 1996). ECMO provides only short-term support, requires intensive nursing management, and is not suitable for ambulatory support. ECMO support is limited to a few weeks; after this time period, multi-system organ failure ensues, probably due to chronic activation of the inflammation that occurs during ECMO support.

3.2 Centrifugal pump VAD

Centrifugal pump systems, such as the Bio-Pump (Medtronic Bio-Medicus, Minneapolis, MN), are the most commonly used form of VAD support for children. Such VADs provide non-pulsatile flow. The centrifugal VAD circuit employs short tubing lengths to connect the pump to the venous and aortic cannulas, which reduces priming volumes compared to ECMO and makes the system easy to maintain(Karl & Horton, 2001). Heparin requirements as well as trauma to blood elements may be decreased with Bio-Pump-based VAD circuits owing to the absence of an oxygenator or venous reservoir. Despite its simplicity and proven track record, the main limitation for the Bio-Pump VAD, like ECMO, is its unsuitability for prolonged support. Thus reported excellent results using the Bio-Pump to support infants and children weighing 6 kg or less (Thuys et al., 1998). Utilizing this system, the authors supported 34 children with median age of 2 months (range 0–8 months) and weight of 3.7 kg (range 1.9–5.98 kg). Of 34 supported, 63 % were successfully separated from VAD support and 31 % of this difficult patient population survived to hospital discharge.

Other reports have described the utility of centrifugal VAD to support the entire spectrum of pediatric cardiac disease (Langley et al., 1998).

3.3 Ventricular assist devices (VADs)

Nonpulsatile centrifugal VADs are used for effective assistance, after a congenital heart surgery of neonates and infants that develop ventricular incompetence. They can be applied especially on patients who will undergo heart transplantation following anomalous origin of the left coronary artery from the pulmonary artery repair or late arterial switch operation and secondary pulmonary hypertension in right heart failure (Del Nido et al., 1999). Discharge survival rate in two studies supported by peroperative centrifugal VAD is around 40 % and have similarities with the usage of ECMO (Duncan et al., 1999; Thuys et al., 1998).

The biggest advantage of centrifugal VAD usage is simplicity of this circulation device. It provides better ventricular decompression than ECMO and does not require oxygenation and requires very low anticoagulation. Although, the usage of biventricular devices on neonates and infants is not realistic, the number of devices is only a few and it requires four cannulas and two pumps. The usage of univentricular VAD is not suitable for patients with resistant respiratory failure, pulmonary hypertension and large intracardiac shunt. It may be used for a few weeks for short term support. The main characteristics of ECMO with centrifugal VAD system are shown on Table 1. There are various devices with long term mechanical support, such as, from paracorporeal VADs to impeller pumps. One of the two paracorporeal VADs, commonly used for neonates and infants is Excor pediatric from Berlin Heart AG and the other is Medos HIA. These are pneumatic devices that work with pulsatile flow. These pumps have different types that can operate on stroke volume under 10 ml for neonates (Merkle et al., 2003; Reinhartz et al., 2002). Thoratec paracorporeal assist devices can be used successfully for adult patients and child patients over 10 years of age, as well (Reinhartz et al., 2001).

Paracorporeal assist devices have been applied on patients with cardiomyopathy or myocarditis for bridging to transplantation. Some patients have been assisted over 100 days, by being extubated and mobilized in the hospital. The usage of these devices for postcardiotomy syndrome is limited and the results are poor. There is a risk of hemorrhagic and thromboembolic stroke in VADs and various neurologic problems may occur (Merkle et al., 2003; Reinhartz et al., 2001).

There are some advanced devices with long term mechanical support in many centers such as DeBakey from Micromed, Jarvik and Incor from Berlin Heart AG that have been produced under the description, impeller axial flow pumps (Song et al., 2003). Today, pediatric version of the DeBakey pump is used and it is still too early to speculate on the success of this pump in pediatric population. Though they have an effective use, only some certain pediatric VADs are approved by FDA (Table 3).

In the United States, several FDA-approved options are available for bridging the patient to recovery and transplantation. These options include the following:

1. Abiomed BVS 5000 circulatory support system (Abiomed, Inc, Danvers, Mass), which is typically used for short-term support
2. Abiomed AB5000 circulatory support system (Abiomed, Inc)
3. Centrimag or Levitronix system (Thoratec, Pleasanton, Calif)
4. Thoratec paracorporeal and intracorporeal LVAD and RVAD (Thoratec)
5. Novacor LVAD (World Heart Inc, Oakland, Calif)
6. HeartMate I LVAD (Thoratec)

Device	Brand	Weight of patient	Pump type
Heart mate LVAD	Thoratec	BSA> 0,7 m^2	Pusher Plate
Thoratec VAD	Thoratec	BSA> 0,7 m^2	Pusher Plate
Abiomed BVS 5000	Abiomed	BSA> 0,7 m^2	Axial
DeBakey VAD	Micro Med Tech.	BSA 0,7-1,5 m^2	Axial
Excor pediatric*	Berlin Heart	> 2,4 kg	Pusher Plate

Table 3. Federal Drug Administration (FDA) approved, ventricular assist devices, suitable for children. (BSA: Body Surface Area, *Can be used for life-threathening conditions, by authorization.)

3.4 Intra-aortic balloon pump (IABP)

The main purpose of intra-aortic balloon pump is to lower the left ventricular afterload of patients with resistant left ventricular failure and to increase coronary perfusion. Balloon is positioned on the descending thoracic aorta. It is filled with helium during diastole, increasing the coronary blood flow. At the beginning of the systole, the balloon is deflated, left ventricular afterload decreases and eventually, cardiac output increases. Although, a sutiable balloon size is available for infants and little children, peripheral vascular complications related to mesenteric extremity ischemia may still occur (Akomea-Agyin et al., 1999). It is hard for the balloon to get in sync on children with high heart rate. There have been many experiences about the usage of IABP on adult patients. However, they are not used in routine practice for infants and little children. IABP may have a role on the treatment of adolescent children with left ventricular failure before placing a different mechanical assist device other than ECMO.

4. Heartmate, Thoratec and the ABIOMED BVS 5000

Several groups have successfully provided mechanical circulatory support for older children utilizing systems designed primarily for adult applications The use of the Heartmate VAD (Thoratec Corp., Pleasanton, CA) in 12 adolescent patients was described. Most of these patients had idiopathic dilated cardiomyopathy. The relatively older age of these patients (range 11–20 years) and larger size (body surface area range 1.4 - 2.2 m^2) allowed the use of this device. As in the adult experience, the majority of children supported by the vented electric model were discharged home with resumption of normal activities (McBride et al., 1999; Korfer at al., 2000).

A number of reports exist describing experience with the Thoratec VAD (Thoratec Corp., Pleasanton, CA) in children. In Reinhartz's review, 101 pediatric patients [median age 13.7 years (range 7-17 years), median weight 54 kg (17–110 kg), median body surface area 1.5 m^2 (range 0.7–2.2 m^2)] had undergone support with the Thoratec VAD worldwide with 66 % survival to hospital discharge (Akomea-Agyin et al., 1999).

Ashton and et al. employed the ABIOMED BVS 5000 (ABIOMED, Inc., Danvers, MA) in four older children. The ABIOMED device was used to provide temporary circulatory support for patients with a body surface area greater than 1,2 m^2 with flows greater than 2 L/ min. A particular limitation to more widespread pediatric application of devices designed primarily for adults can be attributed to low pump rates during support for all but the largest children limiting pump wash-out leading to increased thromboembolic risk (Ashton et al., 1995).

5. MEDOS HIA VAD and the Berlin Heart

The MEDOS HIA VAD (MEDOS Medizintechnik AG, Stolberg, Germany) and the Berlin Heart VAD (Berlin Heart AG, Berlin, Germany) are paracorporeal pulsatile pediatric VAD systems. Because the systems are available in a variety of pump sizes (10–80 ml), they are suitable for the entire age range of pediatric patients including neonates (Shum-Tim et al., 1997). Both are paracorporeal systems that employ pneumatically driven, flexible blood sac pumps, to provide pulsatile flow. Inlet and outlet valves are tri-leaflet and constructed from polyurethane in the smallest versions.

Both the MEDOS and Berlin Heart systems are superior to ECMO in providing moderate to long-term support and preserve the options of bridging to transplantation or recovery for children. Also unlike ECMO, both of these systems allow extubation and ambulation during support with the same effects provided by similar systems designed for adults. Several series have been published describing use of the MEDOS system for pediatric support. Reinhartz reported 64 children supported with the MEDOS HIAVAD, 44 % of whom were supported with the smallest pump sizes with an overall survival of 38 % for patients with available follow-up (Reinhartz et al., 2002). The Berlin Heart VAD has fewer bleeding complications compared to ECMO with decreased blood product utilization during support (Stillert et al., 2004). A recent report showed improving results for infant support in the latest group of patients with survival rates now approaching those achieved in adults (Stiller et al., 2005).

6. The MicroMed DeBakey VAD child (Heart Assist 5)

The DeBakey VAD Child (MicroMed Technology, Inc. Houston, TX) became available for use in 2004. This pediatric device employs the same axial-flow pump used in the adult version with design modifications aimed at reducing the lateral space requirements for device implantation. These design modifications include a shortened inflow cannula with a more acute angle for the inflow tubing, a shortened plastic outflow graft protector and reduced size of the flow probe on the outflow graft. Under the current Humanitarian Device Exemption (HDE), the VAD Child is used to provide temporary left ventricular support as a bridge to cardiac transplantation for children from 5 to 16 years of age with a BSA > 0,7 m^2 and < 1,5 m^2 and is designed to be fully implantable in this size range. Although the clinical experience is still limited, this device has been used successfully in a number of children since its introduction (Morales et al., 2005).

7. Current and future developments pediatric circulatory support devices

The clear need for better means to chronically support the circulation in infants and children with congenital and acquired heart disease resulting in severe heart failure has stimulated recent efforts to develop these much needed devices. The development of these devices is being funded by government agencies, industry, and institutions. The National Heart, Lung, and Blood Institute currently supports the development of pediatric circulatory support devices (Table 4). The program and the devices being developed through NHLBI support are described below;

1. The PediaFlow (University of Pittsburgh; Carnegie Mellon University; Children's Hospital of Pittsburgh; LaunchPoint, LLC; and World Heart Corporation)

2. pCAS (Ension, Inc. University of Louisville; Seare Biomatrix Systems; Fluent, Inc.)
3. Infant- and Child-size Jarvik 2000 (Jarvik Heart, Inc.; University of Maryland Medical Center; Mississippi State University; Whalen Biomedical, Inc.)
4. Penn State PVADs (Penn State University; Minnetronix, Inc.)
5. PediPump (The Children's Hospital at the Cleveland Clinic; The Department of Biomedical Engineering, The Cleveland Clinic Foundation; Foster-Miller Technologies, Inc.)

7.1 Other NHLBI-supported research

1. Pediatric pVAD (CardiacAssist)
2. CardioFlowPQ (Ension)
3. Miniature MagLev VAD (Levitronix)
4. Toddler VAD (Pittsburgh/Carnegie-Mellon University)
5. Fetal Perfusion System (Ension, Inc.)

Device	**Research Institute**	**Pump type**
PediaFlow VAD	University of Pittsburgh	Axial
PediPump	Cleveland Clinic	Axial
PCAS	Ension, Inc, U Louisville	Centrifugal
Pediatric Jarvik 2000	Jarvik Heart, U Maryland	Axial
PVAD	Penn State University	Pneumatic pulsatile pusher plate
RotaFlow	Jostra	Centrifugal
PediVAS	Levitronix	Centrifugal
TinyPump	Tokyo University	Centrifugal
Maglev Pump	Levitronix	Centrifugal (magnetic)
TandemHeart	CardiacAssist, Inc.(Pittsburgh)	Centrifugal

Table 4. Pediatric VADs in development under the NHLBI pediatric circulatory support program (current and future)

8. Patient selection criteria

With the development of new mechanical devices and the increase in ECMO usage, criteria for device usage have improved continuously. Therefore, patient selection cirtieria has become far more important.

- Progression of the disease in spite of high-dose traditional treatment.
- If the purpose is not bridging to transplantation with mechanical support, heart and/or pathophysiology is potentially reversible.
- The hemodynamics is important. Corrective surgery must be conducted and the residual lesion must be defined. Otherwise the presence of an undefined defect may risk the possibility of minimal recuperation and hemodynamic recovery. The detailed postoperative evaluation, ecocardiography, heart catheterization, computerized tomography or magnetic resonance are all of vital importance for the patient.

- The patient must not face with other complications in the intensive care unit. For instance, if there is a cerebral hemorrhage where anticoagulation is contraindicated or if there is a neurologic damage due to hypoxic ischemic encephalopathy, the intensive care support must continue. With a practical point of view, it is not always possible to evaluate the neurological functions of the patient.

In these circumstances, if there is any skepticism about the benefits of the support for the patient, the mechanical support must come to an end, right after neurological function tests. This decision depends on the expectations of the patient's family.

9. The purpose of using mechanical support devices

The main purpose is to provide with suitable physiological environement and time for myocardial recuperation by transferring oxygen to the vital organs, when traditional drug treatment fails. Therefore, stress and myocardial oxygen consumption across the ventricular wall will decrease and adequate coronary perfusion will be provided.

The aim of mechanical cardiac support is to help recover from myocardial failure with effects on heart transplantation and even bridging. Ventricular assist devices and all other new designs are used for pediatric population with the aim of destination therapy.

10. Timing and indications for mechanical support

There are 3 groups for pediatric mechanical cardiac indications:

1. Patients who develop postcardiotomy syndrome
2. Patients with circulatory failure due to myocarditis and cardiomyopathy
3. Patients with heart failure that develops secondary to sepsis pressure (In this section, this will not be discussed with details, but these mechanical support devices have 50-60 % success rate.) (Goldman et al., 1997).

10.1 Postcardiotomy circulatory failure

Mechanical assist devices are sometimes required for pediatric patients with structural heart disease following a heart surgery. Imflammatory response to cardiopulmonary bypass, direct myocardial damage due to surgery, myocardial ischemia due to aortic cross clemp time and reperfusion damage and eventually myocardial dysfunction caused by myocardial exhaustion with postcardiotomy syndrome develop. The repair of anatomic residual lesions that causes circulatory failure is of vital importance. On the other hand, mechanical support indication is low for postcardiotomy patients with malign arrhythmia and resistant pulmonary hypertension.

For the selection of the correct time for starting mechanical support, the risk of organ failure, which depends on the length of time that the patient is going through an invasive treatment like ECMO, must be taken into account. However, ECMO's oxygenation index does not have effective results for preventing a severe disease. With this sensitivity, there are some approaches for the timing of mechanical support in different centers. In spite of suitable vasoactive drug treatment, so many centers activate the postoperative mechanical support with the deterioration of clinical symptoms of oxygen transfer (increase of lactate, decrease of mixed venous oxygen saturation, peripheral cooling, oliguria and other syptoms of end-organ ischemia). In order to avoid organ damage during low cardiac output period, some centers start mechanical support without waiting for the response of drug treatment, due to their concern for myocardial damage that is related to usage of high doses of epinephrine (Reinhartz et al., 2001). Another point of view is that, in spite of the increase of inotropic support (approx. 0,3 microgram/kg/min dose of epinephrine), the mechanical support must be activated due to deteriorating symptoms of low cardiac support. Some centers recommend the usage of VAD in semi effective conditions for postcardiotomy patients who develop severe left ventricular failure after ALCAPA (anomalous left coronary artery from the pulmonary artery) procedure and arterial switch operation (survival rate is 90 %) (Del Nido et al., 1999; Kang et al., 2004).

Some other centers support the usage of VAD, after Norwood Stage 1 operation. Thereby, within 48 hours of the surgery, the patient is protected from the risk of possible neurological disease in later stages by maintaining the brain oxygenation. Another center did not defend mechanical support after Norwood stage 1 operation, in spite of 80 % survival rate that was reported in the very early reviews. While the short term benefit of this support kept out of view, neurological disease must be monitored for long term (Chaturvedi et al., 2004). In another report, while distinguishing a patient with a failure from cardiopulmonary bypass, morbidity and mortality increase, like hemorrhage, was detected (Duncan et al., 1999).

In univentricular and biventricular anatomy, mechanical support indication is related with reversibility potential of myocardial dysfunction, rather than cardiac anatomy as a result. Therefore, patients with single ventricular function may undergo operation, surgical treatment of complex heart lesions would become possible and reversibility potential is maintained with mechanical support indication.

10.2 Circulatory failure due to myocarditis and cardiomyopathy

In popular belief, while heart failure due to cardiymyopathy is a long term disease, myocardial failure on pediatric patients diagnosed with myocarditis, is a fulminant disease that explodes suddenly. Although there are major differences in these two diseases, it is nearly impossible to specify them. It is not always possible to get a diagnosis with myocardial biopsy. It is possible to disconnect the patients with long term cardiomyopathy who require transplantation with signs of acute deterioration, from mechanical support. The importance of the mechanical support and the patients with myocarditis is not rare among some surgeons. Therefore, the mechanical support for these two groups of patients with acute heart failure is suitable. The main purpose of the support is bridging treatment.

The most suitable period for the timing of the mechanical support for these patients is the same with postcardiotomy patients. Development of arryhtmia, intolerance to enteral nutrition and oliguric renal failure are usually bad news. By taking precautions, the wellbeing of the patient must be assured in semi-elective circumstances.

At the end of the first week, if the ventricular function deteriorates, the main purpose must be bridging to transplantation. In this case, long term (monthly) support machines must be considered.

11. Emergency ECMO or extracorporeal cardiopulmonary resuscitation (ECPR)

For patients with, severe problems after a long term cardiac arrest, extracorporeal cardiopulmonary resuscitation (ECPR) is highly recommended for high risk of neurological damage. The succesful results of ECMO placement during cardiac arrest have been reviewed many times recently and have a survival rate of 40 % (Duncan et al., 1998; Morris et al., 2004). The patients who have suffered due to cardiac arrest longer than 60 minutes, continue their neurological life. The results of neurological studies for these patients are important, as these studies prove that they deserve a life in future. The lifesaving effect of ECPR program is that, the surgeon and the surgical nurse are required to have sufficient knowledge, education and cannulation skills for ECMO circulation. So, many centers must have specialists with ECMO experience in their intensive care unit, as an alternative approach. The latest studies show that if crystalloid solution applied with ECMO properly, circulatory support for more than 2 weeks can be maintained (Karimova et al., 2005). ECPR can be improved by this method. It can be stressful to opt for ECMO as a last option for patients with cardiac arrest. With strategic assessments performed under all circumstances, ECMO can be preferred as an early response.

12. Practical point of view for mechanical support

12.1 Cannulation

Veno-arterial ECMO for pediatric patients is performed by inserting cannula into the carotid artery (right carotid artery and right internal jugular vein and femoral vein cannulation) or by surgical procedure of median sternotomy. ECMO cannulation technique for neonates which was introduced by Karl in 1990, allows the preservation of carotid and jugular vessels (Karl et al., 1990). Silastic vessel-loop technique provides adequate hemostasis during ECMO cannulation and allows the reconstruction of the vessels during decannulation.

In patients in whom separation from cardiopulmonary bypass is difficult, further support with ECMO may be useful and aorta and right atrium must be prepped for cannulation. Left atrial vent is placed in some patients where necessary. Postcardiotomoy patients who are undergoing or about to undergo cardiac arrest must be urgently provided with cannulation. If there is enough time and no contraindications, carotid cannulation must be performed. In this way, the risk of infection and bleeding will be minimized.

In an aortic valve failure and impaired left ventricular function, it is important that the left heart must be decompressed. In these circumstances, the pressure of left atrium increases (above 30 mmHg) and lung congestion develops. Left ventricular diastol pressure increases the ventricular wall stress and coronary perfusion deteriorates. Decompression of the left ventricle can be achieved in catheterization laboratory by atrial connection and by direct placement of the left ventricle.

12.2 Bleeding control

Severe bleeding is one of the most important complications of postoperative cardiac ECMO. If the bleeding starts unexpectedly, severe blood transfusion will be required. With the deterioration of the coagulopathy, bleeding increases more.

The following are necessary for the control of postcardiotomy bleeding;

- Improving coagulopathy rapidly (giving thrombocyte transfusion until thrombocytes > 100.000 and cryoprecipitate until fibrinogen > 2 gl/l)
- Keeping activated clotting time (ACT) level between 160-180 seconds (In early stages, it is recommended that activated partial thromboplastin time (aPTT) level must be between 60-80 seconds. The effect of heparin and coagulation ii determined by heparin level, activated factor X and thromboelestogram)
- Application of antifibrinolytic agents (Aprotinin)
- If bleeding continues inspite of improvement of coagulopathy (>10 ml/kg/sec), the thorax might be opened again.

- Opting for carotid cannulation at the neck
- Using the cell-saver device.
- If the bleeding still continues, heparin needs to be cut off within 4-6 hour period until bleeding is stopped (A back-up ECMO circuit must be available at all times).
- In recent years, the usage of recombinant factor VII has been put forward for postcardiotomy patients with resistant bleeding. But routine usage of this treatment is yet to be recommended until the effects are tested by random studies (Pychynska-Pokorska et al., 2004).

13. Mechanical support complications

There are 4 important complications about the usage of cardiac ECMO by ELSO (Extracorporeal Life Support Organization) (Bartlett et al., 1977):

- 30 % bleeding
- Risk of infection (about 30 %)
- Cerebral hemorrhage and infarct (6 % in little children and 12 % in neonates)
- Pump, oxygenation or circulatory failure (10 %)

The most important complications of paracorporeal devices are cerebral symptoms (hemorrhage and thromboembolia) infection and must be diagnosed in the early stages.

14. Efficiency of ECMO

For the assessment, end organ perfusion markers must be checked. Acid-base equilibrium, lactate and mixed venous oxygen saturation, urine output are also put into assessment. The most suitable ECMO flow that enables ventricular improvement is usually 200 ml/kg/sec. The minimum flow that decompresses the ventricle and provides the oxygen transfer may also be favoured.

In oxygen deficiency, hematocrit level must be around 40 % and blood must be separated from oxygenator and adequate oxygen saturation must be maintained. The blood flow can be measured by ultrasonic assessment of the distal section that contains the real blood flow that enables the re-circulation of the patient and which is a bridge to arterial ECMO line. When the real blood flow of the device cannot be measured, bridge to circulation must be clamped and roller pump must be controlled. If symptoms of circulatory failure still occur in spite of these manouvers, there must be an increase in the demand of pump flow for the metabolic needs of the patient. Even at the high flow rate (>200 ml/kg/sec), end-organ circulation may not be maintained. In order to decrease the metabolic requirements of the patient, 34 ^{o}C perfusion might be considered. Vasodilatory drugs can be used to control hypertension while afterload is reduced within necessary intervals. Centrifugal pumps are very important in terms of reducing the afterload and maintaining high volume (Right atrial pressure > 5 mmHg).

15. The use of ECMO for patients with systemic-pulmonary shunt

On patients with Blalock-Taussig shunt (BT shunt) who has undergone Norwood Stage I procedure, the use of VADs is favoured. It can be applied on circumstances where there is no lung problem (Ungerleider et al., 2004). It has been claimed that VAD flow must be at high volume (around 200 ml/kg/minute) in order to provide adequate systemic perfusion and compensate the patients with shunt. On these patients, if ECMO is applied, shunt thrombosis or pulmonary infarction may occur (Jaggers et al., 2000).

The patients who are going through Norwood procedure Stage I with Sano modification, are in need of mechanical support. Here, they require ECMO, rather than VAD. Because, in this physiology, adequate blood flow may not be available in the lungs. In this case, an oxygenator is a must.

16. The follow-up of the patients with mechanical support

There are various physiological approaches; enteral nutrition, a little sedation, the care of the patient's relatives are important. ECMO ventilation must be adjusted according to the resting mode.The tidal volume must be 5-10 ml/kg (highest inspiration pressure to be 25 cmH_2O), PEEP to be 7-10 cmH_2O and ventilation rate to be 15-20/min. In order to avoid pulmonary desaturation, FiO_2 ventilator must be adjusted to 40 %. Unlike ECMO, patients with VAD, full ventilation is compulsory. Antibiotics are not routinely necessary for patients with ECMO. However, daily blood culture monitoring and starting the treatment with the presence of an infection are acceptable approaches.

17. Separation from ECMO (Weaning)

One of the difficulties of ECMO is not being able to determine the clues of ventricular improvement that allows the separation from cardiac mechanical support unit. Practically, the paitent is laid to rest for 48-72 hours, with ECMO support. Later, inotropic perfusiom application (adrenaline or dopamine, combined with milrinone), left atrial vent is clamped and device flow speed is is decreased gradually within two hours until the lowest safe flow is maintained (100-200 ml/minute). However, due to risk of coagulation ECMO flow must not be reduced below this level. If the flow is reduced successfully without risking the hemodynamics, the patient is ready to separate from the ECMO. In this 2-3 hour period, the patient tries to separate from ECMO and then the patient is decannulated. Ecocardiography is used for the evaluation of the ventricular functions. Besides, complications such as, undiagnosed lesions, pulmonary hypertension, akinesia, dyskinesia, pericardial effusion must be re-assessed. If a failure occurs during the separation from ECMO, this is due to inefficiency of the oxygen transfer to the tissues and hemodynamic disturbance. Therefore ECMO support must be re-started immediately and must wait for another 48 hours. This period is best for ventricular recovery and improvement.

18. When to end the mechanical support?

In mechanical support, healing process depends on available pathology. In postcardiotomy patients, myocardial stunning is the basis (Aharon et al., 2001). According to Duncan's suggestion, if signs of ventricular improvement do not occur in this period, the patients must be put on the early transplant list. The timing depends on the organ availability. The separation from mechanical support of the patient who will not undergo transplantation after showing effective signs of cardiac recovery is very important. Survival time with ECMO support is maximum 10 days (Reinhartz et al., 2001; Chaturvedi et al., 2004). In spite of surviving patients who had mechanical support for more than 250 hours, recovery expectancy is highly low for patients who remained under ECMO support for more than 10 days (Morris et al., 2004). After 2 weeks of mechanical support on a patient who is not a transplant candidate, if there are no signs of improvement of ejection fraction, mechanical support must be suspended, according to the practical approach.

One of the most common problems faced with during cardiac ECMO is inefficiency of determining the signs of ventricular recovery. On patients that are separated from mechanical support, traditional echocardiography and oxygen transfer markers are used. In recent years, myocardial tissue Doppler, with its precision to indicate ventricular improvement, is used in evaluating myocardial function (Cheung & Redington, 2004).

Patients with myocarditis can be separated after 2 weeks of mechanical support. These patients will immediately show signs of recovery. If separation from the support (weaning) is inefficient and if the patient is a transplant candidate, the mechanical support must resume as a treatment for bridging to transplantation (Duncan et al., 2001). Besides, there can be limiting factors such as availability of the appropriate mechanical assist device to match the heart of the donor.

In some patients with cardiomyopathy, after 2-3 week period, adequate ventricular improvement of ECMO weaning had been detected. These patients are put into transplant list and a very close follow-up is done (McMahon et al., 2003).

Although there is an increase in the number of pediatric ECMO applications, it is disappointing that the survival rate still remains at 40 % for postcardiotomy patients who have undergone mechanical support (ECLS Registry, 2005). When we take a look at the survival rates, we can see some positive changes, if the support is started in semi-elective circumstances during cardiac arrest. The changes are independent from the usage of mechanical support (Del Nido et al., 1999; Morris et al., 2004). After weaning from assist device, the improvement of low cardiac output that is associated with patients with multi organ failure, neurological complications ensue before ECMO procedure starts (Hintz et al., 2005).

In spite of optimal medical treatment, left ventricular assist devices have not been successful on patients with multi-organ failure. Therefore, with the semi-elective implantation of VAD applications, better results are expected for bridging to transplantation than that of resuscitative implantation. Patients that are expected to undergo left VAD implantation, some cardiac and non-cardiac factors must be analyzed thoroughly. Among these, right heart failure is the most important cause of perioperative mortality. During chronic heart failure, pulmonary vascular resistance (PVR) increases. It usually comes back to normal after transplantation or left ventricular assist device implantation. However, on right ventricular failure that develops severe damage due to left ventricular failure, only left VAD implantation requires biventricular support (Kucukaksu et al., 2002).

Left VAD implantation has both desired and unwelcome effects on right ventricle. The most important effect of left VAD on right ventricle is the decrease of afterload and thus the increase of right ventricular output. However, on 20-50 % of patients who are implanted with left VAD, right ventricular dysfunction is developed. Right VAD must be implanted on patients who have developed right ventricular dysfunction. However, if it is spotted early and inotropic agents, pulmonary vasodilators and phosphodiesterase inhibitors are infused, there might not be a need for right VAD. Therefore the early selection of the patients is clinically important. The patients who require left VAD, while waiting for heart transplant, must be assessed carefully in terms of right ventricular failure (Tarcan et al., 2004).

19. Costs related to ventricular assist device for pediatric use

Historically children with severe heart failure had a significant risk of death while awaiting transplantation. However, the overall survival to transplantation with this strategy is less than 50 %, and the need for ECMO support before transplantation is associated with poorer posttransplant survival (Boucek et al., 2007). The use of VAD therapy to support children with advanced heart failure has increased in the last several years. This increase is related to several factors, including availability of VAD devices for small children and more favorable outcomes in published series. This present study supports the notion that VAD support allows a significant number of children to survive to either heart transplantation or device explantation. The costs of VAD support are considerable greater than $ 500,000 per initial hospitalization and the calculated incremental cost-effectiveness ratio is high even when compared against most other complex pediatric medical interventions. The cost of VAD support in adults has been intensely studied. Investigators have examined both VAD as a bridge to transplantation and VAD as destination. Analyzing VAD as a destination therapy appears somewhat more favorable (Carrier, 2005).

The study assumes that the quality of life after transplant for children who received VAD support is similar to that of other transplant recipients. However, the occurrence of acute neurologic events such as stroke for children supported with VAD may impact later quality of life. In adults stroke occurs in 25% of patients supported for 6 months or longer (Tsukui et al., 2007). Limited data from children would suggest that the risk of stroke is the same if not higher than in adults (Malaisrie et al., 2008). Stroke appears to impair children's social ability along with their neurologic function (Lo et al., 2008). The use of pretransplant VAD has been identified with poorer neurologic function in adults after transplantation (Zierer et al., 2007). In addition, it is assumed that children who undergo VAD implantation have equivalent posttransplant survival to those not receiving VAD support.

Follow-up medical costs are substantial, adding to the overall costs. The costliness of VAD support has been a concern for health-policy officials, engendering much debate. The Canadian government initially limited the use of VAD support, concerned that the cost-effectiveness was unfavorable (McGregor et al., 2000). The costs of postoperative care will be difficult to modify. One strategy might be to discharge a significant number of children from the hospital so that they might be able to wait at home for an available organ. Certainly, adult centers now have a wealth of experience with home VAD management (Oosterom et al., 2007). Previous investigators have shown that home inotropic medication can be administered safely and inexpensively to children awaiting transplantation (Berg et al., 2007). A shorter waiting time would also reduce overall costs. Lastly, the neurodevelopmental outcome of survivors is largely unknown. Children with VAD support before transplantation may have a significantly poorer quality of life than other pediatric transplant recipients. In summary, using VAD support for children with advanced heart failure permits the majority of children to be bridged to heart transplantation. The costs related to this strategy are relatively high and by some standards exceed the threshold for acceptable cost effectiveness. In light of the rapid pace of evolution in VAD technology one hopes that novel approaches can both improve the outcomes and lower the costs associated with VAD support in children.

20. Conclusion

As a summary, the results of patients with myocarditis or cardiomyopathy are highly positive. On patients with myocarditis, if the assist device is used as a treatment for bridging to transplantation, the survival rate is 70 % (Acker, 2001). On pediatric population, treatment for mechanical bridging to transplantation has highly successful results. While survival rate with transplantation is 70-80 %, successful discharge from the hospital is around 70 % (Goldman et al., 2003; Levi et al., 2002). One of the difficulties that relates to the pediatric population for mechanical support team is that, there are more than one ventricular assist devices in use for neonates and children for long term support. The studies of these pediatric cardiac support devices (PediaFlow VDC, PediPump, PCAS, Pediyatrik Jarvik 2000, TinyPump, TandemHeart, RotaFlow) still continue for future use (Table 4). Ideally, these devices have to be implanted on the patient easily. There is a requirement for advanced technology that allows biologically compatible tube systems without the need of systemic anticoagulation. In addition to this, there must be better techniques that evaluate the ventricular function. This will be a guide to the surgeon in decision making about both starting the mechanical support and weaning from it. CE marking shows that the product has met European standards regarding consumer safety, health or environmental requirements and is an abbreviation for Conformité Européenne (European Conformity). There is not price difference of the VAD in Europe and USA. The price of short term devices is between 8-12.000 €, paracorporeal systems 25-50.00 € and axial flow systems (double sided) are about 110.000 €. In recent years, the studies for the manufacture of cardiac support devices in all shapes and sizes still continue to rise. All kind of improvement on this subject is a source of hope for the humankind. The objective for future is to provide permanent solutions.

21. References

Acker, M.A. (2001). Mechanical circulatory support for patients with acute-fulminant myocarditis. *Ann Thorac Surg*; 71:73–6.

Aharon, A.S.; Drinkwater, D.C. Jr; Churchwell, K.B.; Quisling, S.V.; Reddy, V.S. & Taylor, M. (2001). Extracorporeal membrane oxygenation in children after repair of congenital cardiac lesions. *Ann Thorac Surg*; 72:2095–101.

Akomea-Agyin, C.; Kejriwal, N.K.; Franks, R.; Booker, P.D. & Pozzi, M., (1999). Intraaortic balloon pumping in children. *Ann Thorac Surg*; 67:1415–20.

Ashton, R.C.; Oz, M.C. & Michler, R.E. (1995). Left ventricular assist device options in pediatric patients. *ASAIO J*; 41:M277.

Bartlett, R.H.; Gazzaniga, A.B.; Fong S.W.; Jefferies, M.R.; Roohk, H.V. & Haiduc, N. (1977). Extracorporeal membrane oxygenator support for cardiopulmonary failure. *J Thorac Cardiovasc Surg*, 73: 375-86.

Bennett, C.C.; Johnson, A.; Field, D.J. & Elbourne, D. (2001). UK Collaborative ECMO Trial Group. UK collaborative randomised trial of neonatal extracorporeal membrane oxygenation: follow-up to age 4 years. *Lancet*;357:1094–6.

Berg, A.M.; Snell, L. & Mahle, W.T. (2001). Home inotropic therapy in children. *J Heart Lung Transplant*; 26:453–7.

Boucek, M.M.; Aurora, P. & Edwards, L.B. (2007). Registry of the International Society for Heart and Lung Transplantation: tenth official pediatric heart transplantation report. *J Heart Lung Transplant*; 26:796–807.

Carrier, M. (2005). Left ventricular assist device: can Canada afford this? *Can J Cardiol*; 21:1166–8.

Chaturvedi, R.R.; Macrae, D.; Brown, K.L.; Schindler, M.; Smith, E.C. & Davis, K.B. (2004). Cardiac ECMO for biventricular hearts after paediatric open heart surgery. *Heart;* 90: 545–51.

Cheung, M.M.; Redington, A.N., (2004) Assessment of myocardial ventricular function in donor hearts: is isovolumic acceleration measured by tissue Doppler the Holy Grail? *J Heart Lung Transpl* ;23:253–6.

Darling, E.M.; Kaemmer, D.; Lawson, D.S.; Jaggers, J.J. & Ungerleider, R.M. (2001). Use of ECMO without the oxygenator to provide ventricular support after Norwood Stage I procedures. *Ann Thorac Surg;* 71:735–6.

del Nido, P.J.; Armitage, J.M. & Fricker, F.J. (1994). Extracorporeal membrane oxygenation support as a bridge to pediatric heart transplantation. *Circulation;* 90:II66– 9.

del Nido, P.J.; Duncan, B.W.; Mayer, J.E. Jr; Wessel, D.L.; LaPierre, R.A. & Jonas, R.A. (1999). Left ventricular assist device improves survival in children with left ventricular dysfunction after repair of anomalous origin of the left coronary artery from the pulmonary artery. *Ann Thorac Surg* ; 67:169–72.

Delius, R.E.; Bove, E.L. & Meliones, J.N. (1992). Use of extracorporeal life support in patients with congenital heart disease. *Crit Care Med;* 20: 1216– 22.

Duncan, B.W.; Ibrahim, A.E.; Hraska, V.; del Nido, P.J.; Laussen, P.C. & Wessel, D.L. (1998). Use of rapid-deployment extracorporeal membrane oxygenation for the resuscitation of pediatric patients with heart disease after cardiac arrest. *J Thorac Cardiovasc Surg;* 116: 305–11.

Duncan, B.W.; Hraska, V.; Jonas, R.A.; Wessel, D.L.; Del Nido, P.J. & Laussen, P.C. (1999). Mechanical circulatory support in children with cardiac disease. *J Thorac Cardiovasc Surg;* 117: 529–42.

Duncan, B.W., (2001) Extracorporeal membrane oxygenation for children with cardiac disease. In: Duncan, B.W. Mechanical support for cardiac and respiratory failure in pediatric patients. *New York: Marcel Dekker*, 1-20.

Duncan, B.W.; Bohn, D.J.; Atz, A.M.; French, J.W.; Laussen, P.C. & Wessel, D.L. (2001). Mechanical circulatory support for the treatment of children with acute fulminant myocarditis. *J Thorac Cardiovasc Surg;* 122: 440–8.

ECLS Registry Report, (2005), International Summary, July 2005; *Ann Arbor*, MI, USA.

Field, D.; Davis, C.; Elbourne, D., (1996) UK collaborative randomized trial of neonatal extracorporeal membrane oxygenation. *Lancet;* 348: 75–82.

Goldman, A.P.; Kerr, S.J.; Butt, W.; Marsh, M.J.; Murdoch, I.A. & Paul, T. (1997). Extracorporeal support for intractable cardiorespiratory failure due to meningococcal disease. *Lancet;* 349: 466–9.

Goldman, A.P.; Cassidy, J.; de Leval, M.; Haynes, S.; Brown, K. & Whitmore, P. (2003). The waiting game: bridging to paediatric heart transplantation. *Lancet;* 362: 1967–70.

Haines, N.M.; Rycus, P.T.; Zwischenberger, J.B.; Bartlett, R.H. & Undar, A. (2009). Extracorporeal Life Support Registry Report 2008: neonatal and pediatric cardiac cases. *ASAIO, J.;* 55: 111-6.

Hetzer, R.; Loebe, M. & Potapov, E.V. (1998). Circulatory support with pneumatic paracorporeal ventricular assist device in infants and children. *Ann Thorac Surg;* 66: 1498– 506.

Hintz, S.R.; Benitz, W.E.; Colby, C.E.; Sheehan, A.M.; Rycus, P. & Van Meurs, K.P. (2005). Utilization and outcomes of neonatal cardiac extracorporeal life support: 1996–2000. *Pediatr Crit Care Med;* 6: 33–8.

Hunkeler, N.M.; Canter, C.E.; Donze, A. & Spray, T.L. (1992). Extracorporeal life support in cyanotic congenital heart disease before cardiovascular operation. *Am J Cardiol*; 69: 790- 3.

Jaggers, J.J.; Forbess, J.M.; Shah, A.S.; Meliones, J.N.; Kirshbom, P.M. & Miller, C.E. (2000). Extracorporeal membrane oxygenation for infant postcardiotomy support: significance of shunt management. *Ann Thorac Surg*; 69: 1476–83.

Kang, N.; de Leval, M.R.; Elliott, M.; Tsang, V.; Kocyildirim, E. & Sehic, I. (2004). Extending the boundaries of the primary arterial switch operation in patients with transposition of the great arteries and intact ventricular septum. *Circulation*; 110: 123–7.

Karimova, A.; Robertson, A.; Cross, N.; Smith, L.; O'callaghan, M. & Tuleu, C. (2005). A wet-primed ECMO circuit with hollow-fiber membrane oxygenator maintains adequate function for use during CPR after 2 weeks on stand-by. *Crit Care Med*; 33: 1572–6.

Karl, T.R.; Iyer, K.S.; Sano, S. & Mee, R.B, (1990). Infant ECMO cannulation technique allowing preservation of carotid and jugular vessels. *Ann Thorac Surg*; 50:488–9.

Karl, T.R.; Horton, S.B. (2001). Centrifugal pump ventricular assist device in pediatric cardiac surgery. In: Duncan BW, editor. Mechanical support for cardiac and respiratory failure in pediatric patients. *New York' Marcel Dekker*; p. 21–47.

Kato, J.; Seo, T.; Ando, H.; Takagi, H. & Ito, T. (1996). Coronary arterial perfusion during venoarterial extracorporeal membrane oxygenation. *J Thorac Cardiovasc Surg*; 111: 630–6.

Konertz, W.F. (2001). Clinical applications in children of the Medos ventricular assist device. In: Duncan BW. Mechanical support for cardiac and respiratory failure in pediatric patients. *New York: Marcel Dekker*, 269-85.

Korfer, R.; El-Banayosy, A. &Arusoglu, L. (2000). Single-center experience with the Thoratec ventricular assist device. *J Thorac Cardiovasc Surg*; 119: 596–600.

Kucukaksu, S.; Şener, E. & Tasdemir, O. (2002). Bridging to heart transplantation by mechanical assist systems: patient and device selection. *Turkish Journal of Thoracic and Cardiovascular Surgery*; 10: 190–200.

Langley, S.M.; Sheppard, S.B.; Tsang, V.T.; Monro, J.L. & Lamb, R.K. (1998). When is extracorporeal life support worthwhile following repair of congenital heart disease in children? *Eur J Cardiothorac Surg*; 13: 520–5.

Levi, D.; Marelli, D.; Plunkett, M.; Alejos, J., Bresson, J. & Tran, J. (2002). Use of assist devices and ECMO to bridge pediatric patients with cardiomyopathy to transplantation. *J Heart Lung Transpl*; 21:760–70.

Lo, W.; Zamel, K. & Ponnappa, K. (2008). The cost of pediatric stroke care and rehabilitation. *Stroke*; 39: 161–5.

Malaisrie, S.C.; Pelletier, M.P. & Yun, J.J. (2008). Pneumatic paracorporeal ventricular assist device in infants and children: initial Stanford experience. *J Heart Lung Transplant*; 27: 173–7.

McBride, L.R.; Naunheim, K.S.; Fiore, A.C.; Moroney, D.A. & Swartz, M.T. (1999). Clinical experience with 111 Thoratec ventricular assist devices. *Ann Thorac Surg*; 67: 1233–9.

McGregor, M. (2000). Implantable ventricular assist devices: is it time to introduce them in Canada? *Can J Cardiol*; 16: 629–40.

McMahon, A.M.; van Doorn, C.; Burch, M.; Whitmore, P.; Neligan, S. & Rees, P. (2003). Improved early outcome for end-stage dilated cardiomyopathy in children. *J Thorac Cardiovasc Surg*; 126: 1781–7.

Merkle, F.; Boettcher, W.; Stiller, B. & Hetzer, R. (2003). Pulsatile mechanical cardiac assistance in pediatric patients with the Berlin heart ventricular assist device. *J Extracorpor Technol*; 35: 115–20.

Morales, D.L.; Dibardino, D.J. & McKenzie, E.D. (2005). Lessons learned from the first application of the DeBakey VAD Child: an intracorporeal ventricular assist device for children. *J Heart Lung Transplant* ; 24: 331– 7.

Morris, M.C.; Ittenbach, R.F.; Godinez, R.I.; Portnoy, J.D.; Tabbutt, S. & Hanna, B.D. (2004). Risk factors for mortality in 137 pediatric cardiac intensive care unit patients managed with extracorporeal membrane oxygenation. *Crit Care Med*; 32: 1061–9.

Morris, M.C.; Wernovsky, G. & Nadkarni, V.M. (2004). Survival outcomes after extracorporeal cardiopulmonary resuscitation instituted during active chest compression following refractory in hospital pediatric cardiac arrest. *Pediatr Crit Care Med*; 5: 440–6.

Oosterom, A.; de Jonge, N. & Kirkels, J.H. (2007). End-stage heart failure and mechanical circulatory support: feasibility of discharge from hospital. *Neth Heart J*; 15: 45–50.

Pizarro, C.; Davis, D.A.; Healy, R.M.; Kerins, P.J. & Norwood, W.I. (2001). Is there a role for extracorporeal life support after stage I Norwood? *Eur J Cardiothorac Surg*; 19: 294–301.

Pollock, J.C.; Charlton, M.C.; Williams, W.G.; Edmonds, J.F. & Trusler, G.A. (1980). Intraaortic balloon pumping in children. *Ann Thorac Surg*, 29: 522-8.

Pychynska-Pokorska, M.; Moll, J.J.; Krajewski, W. & Jarosik, P. (2004). The use of recombinant coagulation factor VIIa in uncontrolled postoperative bleeding in children undergoing cardiac surgery with cardiopulmonary bypass. *Pediatr Crit Care Med*; 5: 246–50.

Raithel, R.C.; Pennington, D.G.; Boegner, E.; Fiore, A. & Weber, T.R. (1992). Extracorporeal membrane oxygenation in children after cardiac surgery. *Circulation*; 86 (suppl II): II 305–10.

Ratcliffe, M.B.; Bavaria, J.E.; Wenger, R.K.; Bogen, D.K. & Edmunds, L.H. (1991). Left ventricular mechanics of ejecting, postischemic hearts during left ventricular circulatory assistance. *J Thorac Cardiovasc Surg*; 101: 245–55.

Reinhartz, O.; Keith, F.M.; El-Banayosy, A.; McBride, L.R.; Robbins, R.C. & Copeland, J.G. (2001). Multicenter experience with the Thoratec ventricular assist device in children and adolescents. *J Heart Lung Transpl*; 20:439–48.

Reinhartz, O.; Stiller, B.; Eilers, R. & Farrar, D.J. (2002). Current clinical status of pulsatile pediatric circulatory support. *Am Soc Artific Intern Organs J*; 48: 455–9.

Shum-Tim, D.; Duncan, B.W.; Hraska, V.; Friehs, I.; Shin'oka, T. & Jonas, R.A. (1997). Evaluation of a pulsatile pediatric ventricular assist device in an acute right heart failure model. *Ann Thorac Surg*; 64: 1374– 80.

Song, X.; Throckmorton, A.L.; Untaroiu, A.; Patel, S.; Allaire, P.E. & Wood, H.G. (2003). Axial flow blood pumps. *Am Soc Artific Intern Organs J*; 49: 355–64.

Stiller, B.; Lemmer, J. & Merkle, F. (2004). Consumption of blood products during mechanical circulatory support in children: comparison between ECMO and a pulsatile ventricular assist device. *Intensive Care Med*; 30: 1814-20.

Stiller, B.; Weng, Y. & Hubler, M. (2005). Pneumatic pulsatile ventricular assist devices in children under 1 year of age. *Eur J Cardiothorac Surg*; 28: 234–9.

Tarcan, O.; Ozatik, M.A.; Kucuker, S.; Askın, G.; Tufekcioglu, O. & Kucukaksu, S. (2004). The importance and impact of right ventricular functions in left ventricular assist device implantation: case report. *Turkish Journal of Thoracic and Cardiovascular Surgery;* 12: 191–3.

Thuys, C.A.; Mullaly, R.J.; Horton, S.B.; O'Connor, E.B.; Cochrane, A.D. & Brizard, C.P. (1998). Centrifugal ventricular assist in children under 6 kg. *Eur J Cardiothorac Surg;* 13: 130–4.

Tsukui, H.; Abla, A. & Teuteberg, J.J. (2007). Cerebrovascular accidents in patients with a ventricular assist device. *J Thorac Cardiovasc Surg;* 134: 114 –23.

Ungerleider, R.M.; Shen, I.; Burch, G.; Butler, R. & Silberbach, M. (2004). Use of routine ventricular assist following the first stage Norwood procedure. *Cardiol Young;* 14: 61–4.

Veasy, J.G.; Blalock, R.C; Orth, J.L. & Boucek, M.M. (1983) Intraaortic balloon pumping in infants and children. *Circulation;* 1983; 5: 330-3.

Zierer, A.; Melby, S.J. & Voeller, R.K. (2007). Significance of neurologic complications in the modern era of cardiac transplantation. *Ann Thorac Surg;* 83: 1684 -90.